Bonnie Grzesh Pedota

Bon's Year On

my spiritual journey
through panic and anxiety

© Copyright 2006 Bonnie Grzesh Pedota.
All rights reserved. No part of this publication may be reproduced, stored in a retrieval system, or transmitted, in any form or by any means, electronic, mechanical, photocopying, recording, or otherwise, without the written prior permission of the author.

This publication is sold with the understanding that the author and publisher are not engaged in rendering any kind of medical or psychological services in the book. If the reader requires personal medical or psychological assistance or advice, a competent professional should be consulted.

The author and publisher specifically disclaim all responsibility for any liability, loss, or risk, personal or otherwise, which is incurred as a consequence, directly or indirectly, of the use and application of any of the contents of this book.

Note for Librarians: A cataloguing record for this book is available from Library and Archives Canada at www.collectionscanada.ca/amicus/index-e.html
ISBN 1-4120-6439-2

Printed in Victoria, BC, Canada. Printed on paper with minimum 30% recycled fibre. Trafford's print shop runs on "green energy" from solar, wind and other environmentally-friendly power sources.

TRAFFORD
PUBLISHING

Offices in Canada, USA, Ireland and UK

This book was published *on-demand* in cooperation with Trafford Publishing. On-demand publishing is a unique process and service of making a book available for retail sale to the public taking advantage of on-demand manufacturing and Internet marketing. On-demand publishing includes promotions, retail sales, manufacturing, order fulfilment, accounting and collecting royalties on behalf of the author.

Book sales for North America and international:
Trafford Publishing, 6E–2333 Government St.,
Victoria, BC v8t 4p4 CANADA
phone 250 383 6864 (toll-free 1 888 232 4444)
fax 250 383 6804; email to orders@trafford.com

Book sales in Europe:
Trafford Publishing (UK) Limited, 9 Park End Street, 2nd Floor
Oxford, UK ox1 1hh UNITED KINGDOM
phone 44 (0)1865 722 113 (local rate 0845 230 9601)
facsimile 44 (0)1865 722 868; info.uk@trafford.com

Order online at:
trafford.com/05-1350

10 9 8 7 6 5 4

This book is dedicated to all who know the experience of panic disorder. Let us lift the veil of silence. May we proudly stand in our light.

To Kimberley —
Journey on!
Love,
Bonnie

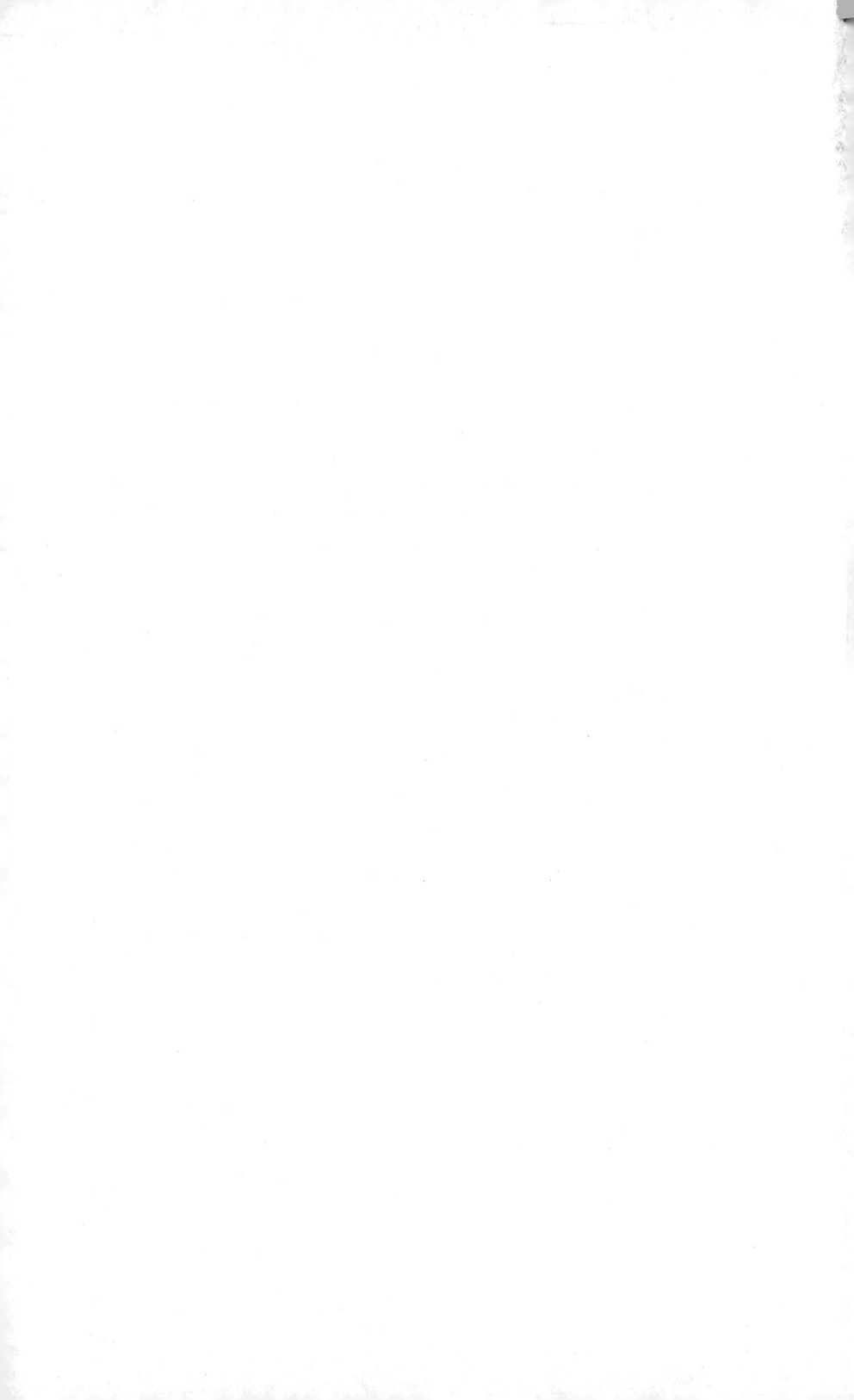

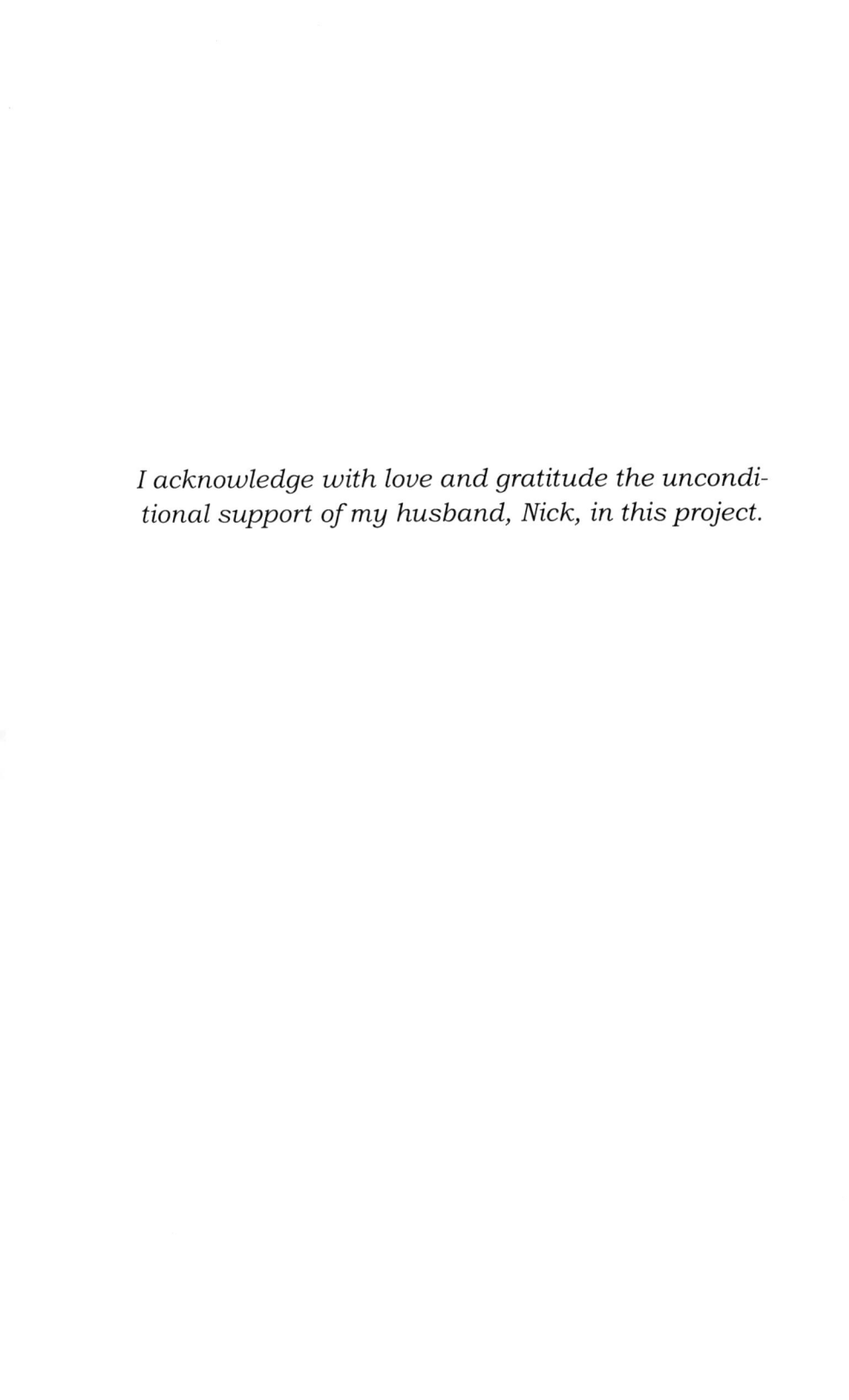

I acknowledge with love and gratitude the unconditional support of my husband, Nick, in this project.

If we have the power to think ourselves into despair then we have the power to think ourselves out of it.

Before I had my first panic attack, there was a world swirling within me that I had little knowledge of. From the day I was born, villages were being built, cities were being run and empires were taking hold.

On the surface, my world looked like one that many of us inhabit. Education was a high priority. Morals such as honesty, loyalty and perseverance were held in high regard. Healthy eating and exercise were encouraged, time with friends and family was valued.

I didn't realize that there were some serious holes in my world's construction. Guilt was a daily if not hourly occurrence. Self-worth was dependent upon the imagined opinions of others. My needs came second, I often said "yes" before I even thought to say "no". I was not entitled to shine.

Recovery from panic disorder came once I was willing to dismantle many parts of my world. I tore down buildings that looked just fine a couple of years before. I asked questions that were not comfortable. I rebuilt one brick at a time.

My new world looks much better. More importantly, it works much better. I watch my thoughts and better recognize the ones that are hurtful. I try to set aside time and space for my spirit. I ask God for help when I am having a tough time with things. I allow myself to fall in love with me.

Contents

Welcome	11
Facts about Panic Disorder	13

♥

Part I: Setting the Stage	**17**
Part II: Panic	**43**
Part III: Recovery	**119**

♥

Appendix A: 10 Minute Relaxation Script	141
Appendix B: Thought Record	145

♥

Annotated References	**147**
Selected Websites	**153**
Thank Yous	**155**

*There is no such thing as a problem
without a gift for you in its hands. You seek problems
because you need their gifts.*
-Richard Bach

Welcome

I am a person just like you – an ambitious, intelligent, "average" middle-class person who thought everything was going okay until it suddenly wasn't. Panic disorder stopped me in my tracks just when I thought life couldn't be better. I didn't see it coming and I sure didn't ask for it. Dealing with it, however, has been the best thing I've ever done for me in my life.

My journey of healing called on my strength (which I discovered I had), my faith (which I found), and the support of those who care (which I sought out).

As absurd as this may sound, I feel lucky that panic disorder became part of my life. Illness has a way of speeding up the healing process, encouraging healing where perhaps we didn't realize there was the need to heal, and then fast-forwarding that process beyond our wildest imagination. I am, without a doubt, a much more whole, reflective, sensitive and spiritual person now than when it all started.

This book is the story of my experience with panic disorder. Here, I share with you the events that led up to my first panic attack, my experience living with panic and anxiety, and the way that I got better. It is not a how-to manual, only you can decide how to heal yourself.

I call this story my *spiritual journey* through panic and anxiety because throughout my healing, I felt as though my spirit was healing alongside my mind and my body.

During the time I suffered from panic disorder, and even before, I kept many journals describing my hopes, feelings, challenges and successes. These journals form the backbone of my story. I have included many journal entries in italics in this book. It is my hope that sharing these intimate parts of my life during the "muck" will help you to feel less alone while you find your way to better health.

Because I believe so strongly in the power of journaling, I have provided the opportunity for you to record your thoughts while you are reading. In Part II, where I describe how panic disorder affected my day-to-day life, you will find prompts to get you thinking about your own anxieties, limiting thoughts, hopes and dreams.

A note: *my* journey of healing from panic disorder did not include drug therapy. While I understand that many people choose to take prescription medication to help them cope with panic attacks and anxiety, I made the choice to heal drug-free. You can certainly meet with lasting success using a combination of approaches. My choice was to talk through my problems with a cognitive behavioural therapist.

If you suffer from panic disorder, and are wondering where the 'old me' went, I have news for you: There is no old me. There is only the 'now me', and the 'amazing me' you will become.

All the best to you on your journey.

Bonnie Pedota
March, 2005

Facts about Panic Disorder

Let's start off with some good news. You are not alone in experiencing an anxiety-related disorder. Not even close. Anxiety is the most prevalent mental health problem for adults in Canada and the United States, according to the Anxiety Disorders Association of Canada[1] and the Anxiety Disorders Association of America.[2] These organizations report that 12.6% of Canadian adults and 13.3% of American adults suffer from some type of anxiety-related disorder. Panic disorder occurs in about 1.3% of the population in Canada, and 1.7% of the population in the United States.

Unfortunately, because mental illness still carries such a strong social stigma, many people suffer in silence. When you are in a room of thirty people, at least two know exactly what you are going through. But you will likely never know. I am certain that most people who suffer from anxiety disorders are embarrassed because I was too. I have a friend who knew about my issues with anxiety. He suffered for over a year, and did not tell me that he also had panic attacks until much later, when he read my book.

Anxiety disorders fall under eleven categories, according to the Diagnostic and Statistical Manual IV (DSM IV) published by the American Psychiatric Association. Panic disorder, agoraphobia, social phobia, generalized anxiety disorder, obsessive-compulsive disorder, and post-traumatic stress disorder are six of these disorders.

---

[1] www.anxietycanada.ca
[2] www.adaa.com

Panic disorder is characterized by panic attacks that happen 'out of the blue'. During a panic attack, you may experience any of the following symptoms:

- Shortness of breath or a feeling of being smothered
- Heart palpitations – pounding heart or accelerated heart rate
- Dizziness, unsteadiness, or faintness
- Trembling or shaking
- Feeling of choking
- Sweating
- Nausea or abdominal distress
- Feeling of unreality – as if you're "not all there"
- Numbness or tingling in hands and feet
- Hot and cold flashes
- Chest pain or discomfort
- Fears of going crazy or losing control
- Fears of dying

In a panic attack, at least four of these symptoms must be present. The other component of panic disorder is the persistent worry about having another panic attack. Both components must be present to be diagnosed with panic disorder.

I have a confession to make. I read these symptoms for panic disorder and recognized them in myself. But I was still in absolute denial that I could have this kind of problem. Finally, two and-a-half years after my first panic attack, I saw a psychologist and he said with absolute certainty that I displayed a 'textbook case' of panic disorder.

I started suffering before the deluge of TV commercials about anti-anxiety and anti-depressant drugs. There was definitely less public awareness about anxiety-related disorders. But the frustrating thing was the lack of awareness even in the professional community. I had seen four therapists and two family physicians, none of whom gave me a diagnosis as clearly as the psychologist finally did.

Whether you decide to work with a psychiatrist, psychologist, or social worker, find someone that specializes in anxiety-related disorders to help you. It will save unwanted frustration, and make your treatment more effective.

.

PART I
SETTING THE STAGE

I believe the journey of healing that used panic disorder as its messenger started well before my first panic attack. Who knows which day that was. It could have been the day I was born. It could have been lifetimes before that.

When looking back at when panic disorder surfaced in my life, there were definitely some minor players that set the stage for a major life change...

♥
Stephen

Stephen D'Amico and I met as teenagers. I was 16 and babysitting for his next-door-neighbor Claire when he wandered into my life. I had been told to expect Stephen to come to the door to pick up some home-made dinner that night. He did, then decided to stay. I was glad to meet a new person, but didn't feel any magic sparks fly. I must have made a good impression on him, however, because he asked me out two days later.

Our courtship was about as exciting as teenage romances go. Stephen, a handsome rebel, went to an all-boys Catholic school and rode a motorcycle. Before our first date, my mother asked, "Where does he go to school?" I either told the truth or pretended I didn't know – either way I knew she wouldn't approve because he wasn't *Jewish*. "We're not getting married!" I argued, thinking it would be one date and that was it. Seven years later, my mother was still shaking her head.

My parents had always envisioned their eldest daughter marrying Jewish, and building a "good Jewish home". Dating Stephen seriously challenged their expectations, and they didn't hesitate to attempt to derail our courtship. My father took issue with the fact that we were seeing too much of each other. My mother lost sleep over the possibility that her future grandchildren might not be Jewish. Unfortunately, none of this mattered to me. I was falling in lust with my first real boyfriend and it was full-steam ahead.

Hormones aside, Stephen and I had little in common. I was studious, he was not. He was a rebel, I was not. I was Jewish, he was not. He was introverted, I was extroverted, and the list went on. For a good four months, though, teenage lust seemed to carry the relationship just fine. Then we had our first argument.

Disagreements between me and Stephen were always recipes for disaster. Thanks to him, we always ended up arguing about *how* we were arguing, rarely getting around to the actual topic of our disagreement. Our first argument was about four months after we met. We were "studying" in the public library, and Stephen implied that he had been hiding something from me. After some humming and hawing, he finally told me: He had been smoking!

Oh my gosh, was I ever furious! I hated cigarette smoke, and he knew that. That evening, I decided to stop by his house to explain how hurt I had been by his confession. Only minutes into our conversation, Stephen was strongly objecting to the *way* I got angry, so I figured it wasn't worth it. I managed to bottle my anger to keep the peace. I later realized that this was something I had learned at home – conflict was scary and to be avoided at all costs. Keeping the peace was very important. It went on this way for several years: Stephen would take issue with the way I got angry (which was never violent *or* confrontational) and I would smooth things over so it didn't get uncomfortable. As a result, we never got many things sorted out in a satisfactory way. Plus, I always felt like I was the one to blame, no matter what the situation was. I would often call up one of my friends after a fight to get an objective view on the situation. Was I nuts? Was I really seeing things the wrong way? How could *he always be right?*

On the day after my senior prom, Stephen broke up with me. He had been ignoring me for weeks, giving me the cold shoulder and not returning my calls. For some reason, Stephen decided to play nice for one night so I could have happy memories of my prom. I'm not sure how he reasoned that would work. The pictures from that night are telling: At the beginning of the night, we're all dressed up and full of expectation, and then by the end of the night, I'm choking back tears, trying to hide my bloodshot eyes.

Figuring I would wash myself of the relationship, I chose to go away to school for my first year of university. I had always dreamed of living away from home, thanks to the *Canby Hall* books I had read when I was young. I have since learned the important distinction between running *away* from something, and running *to* something. Stephen and I broke up around the time final applications were due, and I was definitely running away from the guy that broke my heart. It wasn't that I didn't want to go away – I did. But the main reason for going was to forget him and start a new life at school. I wanted to meet new friends and forget Stephen ever existed. I certainly didn't predict that we would reunite during the first week of school.

Trouble started early, and I see that now. Stephen was jealous of everything, and I suppose he had some reason to be. I was awkwardly straddling the line between brand-new independence and pseudo-married life. While very excited to be at a new school meeting new people and doing new things, I was also heart-heavy, yearning to reunite with my first love. I was excited about going to parties, getting drunk, dancing wildly and being unpredictable for the first time in my life. Stephen caught on in a hurry, a lot sooner than I did.

"YOU DANCED WITH A GUY THAT WASN'T WEARING HIS SHIRT?!?" he demanded. There had been a Halloween drunken-fest in the basement of our co-ed dorm. My friend Keira had come down for the weekend, and we had paid $7 for a bottomless cup of Killer Kool-Aid. It was one of the best parties I'd ever been to. But back in Toronto, I was interrogated:

Stephen: "Do you LIKE him?"
Bonnie: "What do you mean?"
Stephen: "Well, you danced with him and he wasn't wearing his fucking SHIRT!"
Bonnie: "But NOTHING HAPPENED!"
Stephen: "But do you LIKE him?"

I was confused, but more than confused, I was loyal – always loyal. I was not about to give up a two-year relationship over a punk I had just met. I would rather fight to the end: Even if it meant admitting that I did have a crush on that guy (which I did); even if it meant coming home every weekend until the end of the school year (which I did); even if it meant groveling and apologizing until I was blue in the face (which I did); even if it meant allowing myself to be berated, demeaned and treated like garbage (which I did).

The relationship would be saved, and relationship was what I wanted. In *my* mind, there wasn't any other choice.

In retrospect, I suppose I should have broken up with

Stephen the moment I knew he was jealous, the moment I knew he had reason to be. I should have enjoyed my newfound independence, went to wild parties without feeling guilty, and dated different guys. Those are the things you're supposed to do while you're young. To his credit, sometimes Stephen would ask me: "Don't you want some freedom? Don't you want to date and play the field?" I thought he was testing me, but he really meant it and would have let me go if I had said that was what I wanted.

Thankfully, Stephen had become a much different person in the latter half of our seven years together. After four years of being an on-again-off-again jerk, he took me out for dinner one night and explained that he had had a break-down, or rather a "breakthrough". He had realized how horrible he had been to me and to others over the years, and he wanted to start over. He begged my forgiveness with tears in his eyes and pledged a wonderful future together. Most importantly, he thanked me for my unending patience with him.

My reaction at that moment was relief. I felt as though all my patience with him had been for *something*. I had finally gotten through to this guy. My companionship had turned a jerk into a mensch.

Stephen and I enjoyed our last three years together much more than the first four. "He pulled a full 180°," my friend Keira kept saying. Stephen became (and still is) an amazingly spiritual, sensitive, and insightful person. Ironically, after all the trouble we had having a fair fight, he ended up working in the field of conflict resolution. This work brought to light his talent for understanding people. All these wonderful things, however, still didn't mean that we were meant to be together. In February of

1998, I ended the relationship. It was still not letting me shine.

The most important thing I would have changed about the first half of my relationship with Stephen was to better "teach him how to treat me", à la Dr. Phil. I would not have tolerated his insults or his emotional abuse because I would have been strong enough to stand up for myself. I would have said: "If that's the way you're going to treat your girlfriend, and I don't care what she's done, then get yourself another girlfriend!" I would have insisted that he *always* treat me like the decent human being I was. But I didn't teach him all that. I didn't know that I was allowed and indeed obliged to stand up for myself.

♥
Zayda Edek

My maternal grandfather died in June of 1997, and I had to know where he had gone. Not physically, I knew where his body had gone. It made good enough sense to bury someone who had died. I had to know where the person who had lived with us for so long had gone. How could Zayda Edek just no longer *BE?*

Diane Stein's *On Grief and Dying: Understanding the Soul's Journey* picked *me* at a New Age bookstore. It leapt into my hands and I felt incomplete whenever I tried to put it down. Stein's book helped me to understand that people who die do continue living. Their spirits are forever bound up in all the people they loved and interacted with during their lifetime. My grandfather lives on in me, because I knew him. He lives on in all my family members, because he loved so gently, because he was a kind and generous soul.

My grandfather's death got me wondering why death is shrouded in so much mystery, why it is systemically ignored. Why is it not a part of our everyday conversations when it is something we all have in common? Are we so afraid that it will happen to us that we refuse to talk about it?

Another author that helped me through this time was the inspiring and well-known Elisabeth Kübler-Ross. In her book *Death: The Final Stage of Life,* she assures us that death "is an integral part of our lives that gives meaning to human existence. It sets a limit on our time in this life, urging us on to do something productive with that time as long as it is ours to use." Most importantly, "you don't need to nor should you wait until death is at your doorstep before you start to really live."[3]

♥
Yoga

In the summer of '97, I was looking for a good end-of-summer holiday for myself and Stephen. There were usually one or two weeks, before the start of school and after the end of my working at camp, when we could spend some unadulterated relaxation time together.

In Toronto's free health magazine, *Vitality,* I saw an ad for an Ashtanga Yoga Retreat at Shadow Lake Camp in Stouffville, Ontario. Baba Hari Dass, the spiritual leader of the group leading the retreat, would be coming to share wisdom and answer questions. There would be

---
[3] *Death: The Final Stage of Life.* Elisabeth Kübler-Ross. (1975). New York: Touchstone.

opportunities for chanting, meditation, yoga asanas, and a strange new thing for me called "purification". I had had such positive experiences with yoga prior to this, and they offered a good student rate, so I decided to sign both of us up.

Stephen and I had taken yoga classes at university a couple of years before, and were overwhelmed by its calming effects. I missed the first class, so I asked Stephen what he thought, preparing myself for the worst (pain, boredom, etc). "It was just amazing," he reported, and I soon saw it for myself. After the first few classes, I felt so peaceful and calm that speaking seemed superfluous. Life was so much more beautiful and peaceful than I could attempt to describe with words. It was a feeling quite unlike any other.

The schedule at the yoga retreat was quite full. At 5:00 am each morning, we were gently awoken in our dorms by the sound of jingling bells, and requested, though not required, to make our way down to the main hall for chanting, meditation, and purification.

Stephen was far more adventuresome than I was. He attempted all the purification exercises. I was a little more cautious and only felt comfortable trying the purification on the first day.

The purposes of the purifications were to cleanse an interior system. After a brief instruction, we went outside to try for ourselves. On the first day, we were shown how to bend forward and tilt our head to the side, pouring salted water into one nostril, allowing the stream to pass over and through the rear of the nasal cavity to the other nostril, where it exited. It was an uncomfortable feeling at first, but once I got the hang of it, it was fine. Actually, I had never experienced such a clean feeling in my nostrils as I did after that exercise. I could breathe so clearly.

I am sure that the yoga retreat was instrumental in my decision to end my relationship with Stephen less than a year later. The intensive experience with yoga and meditation likely allowed me to tune into my Higher Self. I like to think that my openness to the experience of the retreat let my spirit know that I wasn't afraid to walk in the path of truth.

♥
Sam

The fall after the retreat, Stephen went to work out of town on a conflict resolution job at the University of Waterloo. Though it was low-paying, it was exactly the kind of experience he wanted under his belt. I only saw Stephen on weekends that fall, and it turned out to be the kind of space I needed. As hard as it was to maintain a long-distance relationship, there was some important growth that needed to happen that wouldn't have if he had been home. I would come to see his leaving as perhaps more important for my growth than it was for his.

While Stephen was away, I found myself becoming closer to my friend Sam. Sam and I met a few years before, working together at a summer arts camp. He had been my camp director first, then later my friend.

The way I see it, Sam and I became friends one Saturday morning. I had called him about something work-related, and we ended up talking for well over an hour. At work, we became closer, giggling about silly gossipy things and always connecting through laughter on levels even we were not sure of. It was a grand time.

When we started hanging out together in the fall, it was never less than a five or six hour marathon of Indian food, incense, and inspirational readings. I wasn't sure why I was having such a good time, but I never wanted it to end.

I had convinced Sam to sign up for a yoga class with me at my local community centre. I knew that he would be interested because he had already taken a yoga class with another friend. Mondays became much more bearable that autumn because I knew I would be meeting Sam to go to yoga at the end of the day. We often stopped at a nearby deli to scarf down potato bourikas and spinach pies before class. I didn't want to admit it to myself, but it was a major crush in the making.

Journal Entry – Nov. 17/97
…I think it's time to re-think and re-group. I am getting too carried away with Sam. I know. It's just that I get along so well with him – I feel good when we talk – we laugh together and connect on so many levels. But I guess I'm getting too into this – letting myself be spread too thin. Forgetting about Stephen when I should be spending all my time with him. <u>I'M SO CONFUSED</u>.

Nov. 18/97 (1 am)
B-day officially over – still pissed that Steve sort of ruined it. But Sam totally cheered me up – gave me presents and a really nice card – with a poem and an inspirational quotes book and he kept on saying "Happy Birthday" in Yoga – he totally made me feel good. Ironic – the guy that's my friend makes me feel better than my boyfriend. (and he called and left a message on my

machine while I was out for dessert – just so I would have another happy birthday message) What a guy. I don't know what's happening here. Help. Follow your heart or follow your head – or not that simple.

Here's the truth – I feel good when I'm around Sam – we have the best time. I don't know why I feel like I'm becoming attracted to him. But I look forward to seeing him, and it feels wrong because of Stephen. WRONG. But right. Help.

Nov. 18/97 (11 pm)

...I am <u>SO</u> confused. I love spending time with Sam, and I find myself not wanting it to end. I feel like I'm falling for him, but I can't be – but I am. I feel so guilty. I cry. Sam and I went to the herbalist and then to Tandoori House and then to Yorkdale and why did I keep thinking 'I don't want this time to end'? I am in trouble. Huge. You can't love two people at once. You can.

It's just not supposed to happen because it's not acceptable. Part of me knows I have to tell Stephen what's going on in my head. Part of me says I'd better forget about Sam as fast as I can. The better part says 'why would you throw away something as wonderful as this'.

Nov 19/97

...I know I have to – and can – tell Stephen about Sam, and about what is happening to me. I must. Because I feel like it's made me look at my relationship with him. I was reading Soap Opera Digest – about how Carrie and Austin have been together since they were teens, and Mike is this older guy who she really loves but doesn't know it yet. And I'm thinking – Oh my God – this is my life – here in Soap Opera Digest which I never read, but my mother bought for me for obviously this reason (maybe).

Stephen and I were never friends first. We rushed into this head on, and it is the exact opposite of what happened with Sam and me. Sam and I were friends first – this friendship that sort of took off from nowhere but exploded into fireworks. We connected – we did – we do...

...Help. This is not supposed to happen. (or maybe it is – it is necessary to look at it in order to see it for what it is). All in the process. Of growth and all that. The year of growth. That is what this is for me. It has been good – I hope it continues to be.

For my 24th birthday, I decided I was going to have a "Japanese Dinner Party" at my parents' place. I invited ten of my closest friends to come and eat miso soup, sushi, spicy eggplant, and sip jasmine tea. Stephen had come in for the weekend from his out-of-town job. Saturday morning, we ran around picking up all the essential ingredients before we started preparing.

I started to have a horrible sinking feeling in my stomach. *I didn't want to be around him.* He didn't seem interesting enough. I wanted to be spending the day with Sam. Stephen was the last person I want to do errands with. Shush, shush, shush, I told my conscience.

Nov 23/97
Wow! What a week. I had a dinner party last night for 10 people!! What was I thinking? It went great, though. Sit-down, 3 courses and everything. With a lot of help from Steve and Keira! Talk about good karma, though. It was amazing what people wrote in my cards! Since I've been sending out all this positive energy lately, giving compliments, being true to myself, being honest, etc, I think it might have all come back to me – like throwing

a ball against the wall and it comes back to you or dropping a rock in the ocean, and all the ripples coming out of it. Everyone (just about) wrote about how I'm such a great person and how they're glad to be friends with me – I was <u>SO</u> touched! And all the gifts were so uniquely <u>me</u>. Books about growth and healing and candles – my goodness people know me!

And Stephen and I had <u>the best</u> talk after everyone left, about how I, with all this Sam stuff, have been forced to turn our relationship on its head and question it. And how I need space to figure this out – how I need to know I need him and want him, but I have to stand on my own. I started the conversation with the strange discovery that every time Stephen leaves, I <u>GROW</u>. And that made me sad. Why is that the way it is? It's sad. I told him I still feel like I'm trying to be someone when I'm with him – and I'm not happy when that happens – it's dissonant. And (I just realized) that Steve's going away and my growth also goes along with me being closer to Sam! Why is Sam so instrumental in my growth? And why does it only happen when Stephen leaves? Because I feel I can't grow with Sam when Steve is here? And what is it about Sam that allows me to grow (did I ask this already?) That I feel like I am being myself??

The thing is that I feel like I need time away from Stephen. For healthy reasons. I have never seen other people – never dated. And I'm beginning to feel like I'm missing out. Stephen talked about 'The 7-year itch', which I don't like the sounds of at all, because I feel "pegged" – like it happens to everyone, and I'll get over it. And the thing is that this is <u>SUCH</u> an individual experience that that label bugs the hell out of me.

… What I love about what Sam has (unintentionally) done for me is that it has forced me to question my rela-

tionship with Stephen and not just BE in it, but reflect on it, and know that it's the right thing, or that maybe it's not. But the worst thing of all would have been not to have questioned it. Like in university they teach you to question everything – not believe everything you read. I feel good about this – like when (or if) I realize that I should be with Stephen, it will be for real – and I will be with him for all the right reasons. But at the same time it scares the shit out of me – not being with him. But at the same time, nothing has ever made this much sense to me. WEIRD.

This has been the month of me. And nothing has felt better. I hope I keep on feeling this good and making others feel good for a long time to come. I feel changed, and good. Very good. Right. Keep faith that the right thing will happen if I believe in myself and love myself.

Nov 27/97

Well, it's been since Monday (or Saturday) that I have been taking this 'break' from Stephen. It has been trying. Sometimes I'm high as a kite, and then sometimes reality kicks in and I'm low and depressed. I sometimes forget about why I'm doing this. But I'm doing this for me. For loving myself. For being okay with me. I have figured out, through talking with Keira, why I feel good when I'm with Sam. It's because he clings to my every word – he listens with everything, and the message is – 'You are important. You are great. I like you for who you are, and what you say to me.' And that is attractive. To have someone give you those affirming messages is so amazing. And that's why I am 'attracted' to him. And why I was driven to spend as much time as possible with him – because I felt good. Affirmed. Validated. And it's funny, but now that I've realized that, I don't feel like I NEED him that much

– like I want to spend all my time with him. Now that I've figured that out it's a whole new game for some reason. I am not making these unrealistic expectations of him. I am back in reality – he is a very busy and very TIRED person, and not only do I have to respect that, but I have to be OKAY with that. Okay without him. Okay with him being ONE of my friends, and not necessarily my <u>best</u> friend. Because I have Kate and I have Keira too. And they help me too. That's probably why I was driven to spend time with Kate at the beginning of the year – because she made me feel good about me. I am thankful that these people have entered my life to help me realize these things about myself. I need to realize these things before I marry Stephen (or anyone). It's okay to not be with him for a bit. Until I am ready to be with him again for good. Or not. But it's OKAY.

Stephen and I took our break. Then a couple of weeks later, we got back together. I can't remember why we did. I suppose it was just easier than having to deal with the emotional messiness that is the end of a long-term relationship. But deep down inside I knew that I had settled. I was waiting for a great boulder to fall from the sky and smite me down because I wasn't being 100% true to myself. I couldn't figure out why the sidewalks I was walking that month didn't just drop off at the end. How could the world go on spinning when I had made a choice that I knew wasn't in my best interest?

♥
Reiki

One of the reasons that I love Reiki is that it is available to everyone: young and old, healthy and sick, tall and short, big or little. Reiki does not attach itself to a particular religion. Healing occurs when people called 'channels' place their hands in set positions on the receiver's body, and then proceed to different positions in a specific order. Gentle music is often played to induce a state of relaxation, but this is not necessary. Healers and people who are receiving 'hands-on' report a variety of sensations during a session. These can include heat, cold, tingling and others.

Reiki (pronounced Ray-Kee) "is a method of natural healing based on the application of Universal Life Force Energy (the name literally means Universal Life Force Energy)." [4] The basic principles of Reiki are:

> *Just for today, do not worry.*
> *Just for today, do not anger.*
> *Honor your parents, teachers, and elders.*
> *Earn your living honestly.*
> *Show gratitude to everything.*
> -Dr. Mikao Usui

The first time I received Reiki, I was amazed. I felt a lot of heat coming from the hands of my channels. I was intrigued. I wanted to know what the channels were picking up while they were standing there so patiently with their hot hands, placing them in the prescribed positions.

After the session, I felt physically balanced. I felt symmetrical, like my left and right sides were even, with a line running down the middle.

The next morning I woke up absolutely high on life. To this day, I have never experienced anything as

---
[4] http://reiki.7gen.com/

spiritually powerful as the impact of that first Reiki session:

> *May 12, 1997*
> *I feel as though a whole life has opened up – a vision that I don't want to leave – ever. Living life to the fullest, and making life happen, rather than letting things happen. I feel so in-touch. With me, with the future, even. Although I can't predict the future, I know that the things I do are all for a reason. I believe the Celestine Prophecy idea that when you are in touch with yourself and your energy, you can direct and understand the coincidences in your life.*

My mother signed up and paid for me to take my Reiki I certification because she had benefited from it so much herself. She had taken her Reiki I certification when her father had been dying in the intensive care unit. During the evenings when she would visit her father, Reiki empowered her to feel she could help him in some way.

Because of the impact of my first Reiki experience, it was not difficult to sell me on taking the Reiki I class. The timing was eerie, now that I look back. I had just started communicating with my friend Nick, whom I hadn't spoken to in three years. We were mending a friendship that I had ended because I was uncomfortable with Nick's feelings for me. Reiki assisted in the mending of that friendship beyond my wildest imagination.

Our instructors, Denise and John Crundall from Australia, were greatly admired by the people in our Reiki centre in Toronto for their work around the world teaching and delivering Reiki. Denise did most of the lecturing when I took the course, and I just sucked up everything she was saying. She shared personal stories of healing with Reiki, including those about her own family. She spoke of New Age principals, ("Love yourself enough to love another more"), and about the metaphysical causes of illness – for example, the onset of asthma reflects unhealed grieving from the past. I took pages and pages of notes, incredibly excited to learn new perspectives on illness and on healing.

At the end of the weekend, our training was complete, and we were officially Reiki Channels. Reiki legend holds that twenty-one days after you receive your Reiki I 'fine tuning', something major will shift in your life. I never would have guessed what was in store.

♥
Nick

Nick Pedota and I were great friends, so great that I hadn't spoken to him in three years. We were meant to be together, but I wasn't so forgiving back in 1995 when he professed his love for me while I was still involved with Stephen. Instead, I chose the path of fear and cut things off between us.

Fast forward to January of 1998. Nick was working in California (or so I thought) when I finally decided to let bygones be bygones. Talking to someone thousands of miles away couldn't be that threatening, I reasoned. Plus, two months had passed since the emotional roller coaster involving Sam, and I figured I was ready to face anything. I missed Nick, and I didn't want to throw away a great friendship because of fear. I had started reading Marianne Williamson's *A Return To Love*, and was fueled by her insights and wisdom. I bravely placed

Setting the Stage

the call to Nick's parents' place and was surprised to find out that he had moved back to Toronto.

Our first conversation and outing were spectacular. Nick was what he had always been: generous, kind, and easy to talk to. It took less than a moment for the heavens to celebrate us rebuilding our friendship.

Jan 9/98

Holy cow! Nick and I <u>totally</u> reconnected. We talked Monday night (for the first time in 3 years) and we are totally at similar points in our life – we have both done a whole lot of growing up. He is a totally different person and yet the same incredible guy I got along with so well so long ago. SO COOL. Amazing.

...It's just real nice to have him back in my life. I thought about him a lot, obviously because he means a lot to me. It's a friendship my life is richer for having. Sort of like coming home.

I was ecstatic and elated, but within two weeks Nick was throwing up the red flags, afraid that he was falling for me again, afraid that I wasn't. *A Return to Love* in hand, I reassured him that I was going to stick it through this time. Williamson says: "In every relationship, in every moment we teach either love or fear."[5] I wasn't going to let my fear of my feelings for Nick (or his for me) stand in the way of a great friendship this time, whether I had a boyfriend or not – and I still did. I was being given a second chance, and I wasn't going to blow it this time.

Then something shifted. I realized I was becoming attracted to Nick. "Magnetically attracted," I wrote in my journal, along with all kinds of names I called my-

---

[5] *A Return to Love*. Marianne Willliamson. (1996). Canada: HarperCollins.

self: "Incomplete without a man", "clingy", "dependent". I was so unwilling to accept the fact that I had feelings for him, that I was willing to make myself the enemy. I turned things on their head that never needed to be. I decided that I talk too much, then I decided that's just who I am. I was all messed up all over again.

Williamson writes: "Real work can only occur in the presence of rigorous honesty,"[6] and that was my motto. I was going to be honest with Nick, and I was going to be honest with Stephen. That was a tough month. I couldn't understand why I felt the need to talk to or be around Nick all the time. Since Stephen was still working out of town, I figured I was trying to fill some void that Stephen had left by being away. Calling myself names did little to explain why I felt so good around Nick and some other special friends and less good when I was with Stephen – and really guilty for it.

During this time, I took Marianne Williamson up on a suggestion. She wrote that it's alright – if you're stuck – to ask for a miracle. When you can't see a way out on your own, it's okay and right to ask God to intervene.

So I did. I sat in a subway station waiting for a friend, and from the bottom of my confused, miserable heart asked God for a miracle. And wouldn't you know it, God delivered in less than two weeks.

I was talking to my girlfriend Kate when it hit me. Being with people who make you feel like a great human being, just by being yourself, is a good thing. In fact, that's probably the kind of person you want to be with for the rest of your life.

---

[6] *A Return to Love*. Marianne Willliamson. (1996). Canada: HarperCollins.

Setting the Stage

Feb. 5, 1998

I finally got it. I am not a bad person or a bad girlfriend. I just deserve better. I deserve the happiness I have with Nick (& Sam & Kate & my really great friends) with the man I choose to live my life with. Nothing less. It's about being me and being proud to be me. It's about the chemistry between two people that brings out the best in me, and makes me think, "Yeah, I am cool." And I don't get that with Stephen. And nothing I do or say is going to put it there. Nothing. So all I can say is I gave it my best shot, and I'm glad I realized this before I made the mistake of marrying someone who makes me feel okay, but not amazing. Because that's what I am. Amazing. And one day, some really good-looking man is going to come along and make me feel that great. Because Nick does it. And Sam does it. And Kate does it. So it can happen again. And it will. I don't deserve anything less. I love Stephen more than anything, but it's time to step out. For me. ♥♥♥

Nick and I got together three days after I broke up with Stephen. When I took his hand in mine for the first time, all was right in the world. We talked and hugged all night long, and during that time I felt like all the nasty demons I had ever accrued were magically falling one by one from my body. That negativity, particularly what I had experienced in the early part of my relationship with Stephen, was no match for the love that Nick and I shared. God and his angels blessed us in ways I never imagined. I left Nick's house early the next morning feeling lighter than I had ever felt in my life.

♥
Graduate School

I was in the second year of my master's degree when Nick and I got together. While my personal life was proceeding in leaps and bounds, my professional life was in the gutter. I was trying desperately to feign interest in boring courses while attempting to write a thesis for a supervisor that was on sabbatical. Being a graduate student depressed me, and after writing two unsubmitted thesis proposals, I realized I was going to walk away. It was the classic "high achiever" meets "lack of motivation" nightmare:

March 13/98
...If my relationship with Nick went so right, why can't I get the other parts of my life in order? Like school. And work. But especially school. What a fucking toll it's taking on me. I'm gaining a shit load of weight because it depresses the hell out of me. That makes me so mad – that something can have this much control over me. I don't deserve this. I deserve me first. My life got better before when I took control. Made active decisions that said "Me first!!". So I don't know if I can do that here. I'm a bit of a chicken shit because I don't want to leave my degree undone. It's not like me to not finish what I started. But maybe this is the new me. The one that says "Me first. All you other losers later." (Meaning academic institutions or any other entity that undermines Bonnie's happiness for even a second.) So maybe I'll take that leave this summer. Get this fucking thing the hell out of my life for just a little while, and see how that feels....
The important thing is that I stop killing myself. I don't

deserve it. No one does. So I choose me again. It feels great. I should feel great in no time. By keep on choosing me. Above all else. The rest will fall into place. Like it did with Nick. And now it will again, with any luck. God it takes a lot of courage to be happy. To say 'me first'. It's easy to forget. But not when you ask for help. Thank God for this divinity he shows when we ask to see it. Thanks.

PART II
PANIC

Panic

♥

I had my first full-blown panic attack when I was 24 years old. Four months earlier, I had ended a seven-year relationship and started a new one with my soul-mate. Six weeks earlier, I had walked away from an unfinished Master's degree because research was making me miserable.

It was the day before Father's Day, 1998, and Nick and I were ending a fabulous three-week tour of Western Europe. Nick thought it would be perfect to end our trip with an evening outing to Montmartre, escorted by our Parisian friends Catherine and Xavier:

June 21/98

...Well, we never made it to Montmartre because something happened in the car on the way there. I had had a mild headache from about 5:00 on. Nick and I had lay down for a nap and ever since then, I felt groggy and a bit headachy. So in the car, I'm suddenly feeling like this headache could get the better of me – could knock me right out. And it almost did. All of a sudden, I felt like I couldn't breathe. We asked Xavier to pull over for some water, which he did, but then I started feeling worse – like I couldn't breathe at all – and my fingers then my arms and legs started getting all tingly. Then I really started panicking – I thought I was going to die because of my loss of breath. I thought if I pass out (which was seeming inevitable), then that's it! Nick was also in panic mode because I kept on saying 'I don't know what's happening!'. Finally Catherine and Xavier came back and rushed me to the hospital. We actually pulled up beside a cop, who (upon Catherine's request) escorted us to the hospital with sirens on! Hopefully that will be the last

time I'll need a police (or any) siren escort! Anyhow, at the hospital I was still freaking out because I was all tingly – arms, legs, and front of body. This nurse saw me right away – took my temperature and then asked everyone to leave because she was going to do a cardiogram. I told her I was scared (in French!) and she kept telling me to relax but that seemed impossible. Finally, she let the others back in. The doctor came (a woman, really nice!) and started asking me questions – medical history and stuff. Slowly, things were starting to get better. I guess I stopped hyperventilating a bit. She told me it was likely the heat (she said it gets her too sometimes) and that I should drink 1 L of water and then go to bed. That's what I did, but not before a good cry because that was scary shit. I've never been so scared (health wise) before – the whole passing out (or feeling like I was going to) freaked me out to no end.

On that day, I had no idea that I had suffered my first full-fledged panic attack. In the weeks that followed, I became convinced that many other things could have happened. I was more confused and scared than I had ever been in my life. How could I be sure it wouldn't happen again?

♥
Camp

I returned to normal life for a short period after our return from Europe. That summer, I was working as a Camp Director for a city-run arts camp. Achieving this position was an affirmation of all the hard work I had put in as a counsellor and instructor for nine consecutive summers with the Parks and Recreation

Panic

department. Panic and anxiety were about to take me in an entirely different direction.

When my Assistant Director and I were finishing up some things before the start of training week, I casually recounted my story about not being able to breathe in Paris. "You're not going to believe this," I began casually, while inside I was still highly traumatized over the event. I relayed my amazement at my quick return to normalcy.

After eating lunch one day during our training week, my heart started pounding uncomfortably. What was going on? I became scared that I was going to pass out. I realized that I was not going to make it through the next activity so I excused myself and rushed over to my herbalist, Diego.

Although Diego was just down the street, I arrived in a panic. After waiting a few minutes, I told the receptionist that I thought I was going to pass out. She informed Diego of the seriousness of my condition, and tried to calm me down. She suggested I put my head between my knees, but that made things even worse.

"Oh my!" he said when he finally saw me, "You have a very bad infection in the heart and lungs!" My fear nearly had me in tears, but I knew that if I started to cry, I would feel worse. Diego performed some energy healing for twenty minutes, gave me some herbs to take home, and then let me rest in his back room. As I lay there, my heart was still pounding, and I still felt like I was on the verge of passing out. I thought about calling out to Diego for help, but I didn't.

About twenty minutes later, Nick showed up to escort me home. When I stood up to leave, I did feel a little bit better. I paid for the herbs and Nick followed me home in his car. We stopped at the mall to do an errand, and then my heart started pounding again. We left my car in the parking lot and Nick drove me home.

At home, I lay in bed with my heart pounding for what felt like hours. Nick had picked up the pictures from our trip to Europe, and I didn't even feel like I could sit up to look at them. That was highly unusual because of my love for pictures.

I didn't return to work for the rest of the week, and feared whether I would feel well enough to be there for the opening day. I felt like I had disappointed everyone, especially my Assistant Director, by getting this mysterious and debilitating illness. I felt like I was bailing out on training week, something I had looked forward to.

Though I was still feeling dizzy and disoriented, I forced myself to show up for opening day. Fear figured prominently into that day and into the following weeks. I stumbled my way through the first two-week session, though I really didn't feel up to doing the job. My symptoms returned in waves. Sometimes I'd feel almost okay, then when I would go out into the heat and humidity, I'd feel like I couldn't breathe and I'd start to panic.

Near the end of the first two-week session, my supervisor became concerned. She suggested I take the rest of the week off, and make an appointment with my family physician.

My family physician found nothing physically wrong with me, but when my symptoms didn't improve, I made a second appointment a week later. My doctor then diagnosed an inner ear infection because of my constant dizziness. When I asked her why my heart was pounding, she explained that that was the heart's response to the presence of infection in the body. My herbalist, on the other hand, said that I didn't have an inner-ear infection, but a lung infection, and later a problem with my liver. He gave me amino acids to strengthen the muscles in my lungs, and desiccated liver tablets to strengthen my liver. The shortcomings of the Western medical model were shining through: a thorough underestimation of the contribution of mind and spirit to overall health. It wasn't my physical body that needed healing that summer, but that didn't mean I wasn't sick.

At the end of the first two-week session of camp, Nick whisked me away to a bed and breakfast in Bracebridge, just two hours away. It was meant as a retreat from the stresses of the city, but I carried with me whatever it was that needed to heal.

Leaving the city, I felt weak and dizzy. Nick had reserved us a private cabin outside of the main B&B which was brand new and very nice. However, soon after settling in, I felt another attack coming on. I felt like I couldn't breathe. My fingers got tingly, then my arms. I was so scared. I tried my best to breathe, but it felt like I was sucking air in through a straw. There was nothing Nick could do, so I just told him to lie still until I felt better.

I could barely eat the next morning at breakfast. I felt bad that Nick had spent so much money on the cabin and I wasn't even eating.

Fear is an excellent master, but not a great companion. I was afraid of so much that summer, it's amazing that I didn't just fall off the earth. I was afraid that I was going to die. I was afraid that I was going to embarrass myself with my 'problem'. I was afraid that other people thought I was a flake, because I missed so many days of work. I couldn't go into a public place without feeling dizzy and overwhelmed, or walk to the end of my street without feeling out of breath. I often needed to use a pad of paper and pen to get a message out because I would feel choked and panicky when speaking. Nick had to call my friend Sam once to 'babysit' me because I was bored, but I would only allow someone who understood my unique condition to come over.

My progress was so slow it often brought me to tears. I would wake up in the morning feeling fine, so I would start to work on something like cleaning out my closet or desk drawers. But before I knew it, I felt like I couldn't breathe, and I was forced to sit on the couch in front of the TV until I felt like I could move again. It was paralyzing.

I was forced to quit my job as Camp Director because I was not physically capable of doing the job. It broke my heart, but God had other plans for me. My spiritual journey would take precedence over my physical journey.

♥

Over the span of two years, I would try a large number of therapies to help cure my condition. Reiki, Shiatsu, energy work, acupuncture, massage therapy, healing prayer, psychics, an herbalist... you name it, I tried it. None of these seemed to get to the root of the problem. At best, they helped for a short amount of time. I do not dismiss these therapies as ineffective; in fact I still keep some of them in my 'maintenance toolkit'. However, none of them were effective at treating my panic and anxiety in a way that was long-lasting.

♥
The Year On

My dissatisfaction with graduate school had got me thinking about what I would enjoy more. In a meditation, I realized that I loved being with kids more than anything. I applied, was accepted and prepared to go to teachers' college in the fall.

Unfortunately, when the summer of my first panic attacks came to an end and I wasn't feeling significantly better, I realized that I was going to have to postpone going to teachers' college to recuperate and take stock.

I sat at the kitchen table with my mother at the end of August, crying because it was so hard for me to admit defeat; crying because I felt like I was asking her permission to go against the grain and take a year off from my studies; crying because I realized I was going to choose me again. Perhaps going to school for the twenty-first consecutive year was not in my best interest. I felt liberated, empowered, and lucky because she supported my decision.

Soon, I decided that I wasn't taking a "year off" from school. I was taking a "Year ON" for Bonnie. I had never done that...never traveled alone, never taken a break from school, never explored my likes, dislikes, and spirit in an intense way.

I went downtown and bought a journal that I had seen a couple of weeks before. It was very unique. The pages were yellow and looked like the homemade paper I used to make at day camp. The cover was textured and had two strings hanging with brown beads tied on.

Bon's Year On

Sept. 16, 1998

This year began as a 'year off'. However, I soon realized that nothing could be further from the truth. This is a year on. A year of exploring me. Of enjoying life, of doing the things I enjoy doing, and not feeling guilty about doing them.

This year is also a search. For my true creative genius, whatever that may be.

Best of all, this year is a journey without an end in sight. A journey built on faith. That once I discover the true creative genius within me, it will carry me in my life – providing for me as I provide for myself.

On the first page, I welcomed inspiration in any form. I wrote these words in a spiral:
ANYTHING.
A DREAM.
A THOUGHT.
A WEDDING PLAN.
A MEDITATION.
A SHOPPING LIST.
A 'THINGS-TO-DO' LIST.
A PICTURE.
A DOODLE.
A SCRATCH.
A SONG.
A POEM?
A VERSE.
A SELF-PORTRAIT.
A LIST OF FRIENDS.
A PLAN.
A STREAM-OF-CONSCIOUSNESS.
A RHYME.
A PHOTOGRAPH.

A RECEIPT.
A STICKER.
A TATOO.
A SCENT.
A STAIN.
A SMUDGE.
A BRIDAL PARTY.
A LIST OF FAVOURITES.
A LIST OF THINGS I WANT TO DO.
A TRIANGLE.
ANYTHING ME.
☺

Success, as they say, is 5% inspiration and 95% perspiration. Though there would be a long journey ahead, I was off to a good start.

What kinds of possibilities have anxiety and/or panic disorder opened up for you? How have you grown since you started suffering?

♥
The First Step

During the summer I had spent home sick, Stephen visited me once. He wanted to help me out in any way he could, so he offered me a business card for a psychotherapist named Dr. Solomon. A friend of his highly recommended him. At this stage I was willing to try anything.

Dr. S. had been a family physician for many years, and had become frustrated with the number of health problems walking through his door that didn't have biological origins. He realized that these patients could be better helped with a good dose of psychoanalysis, so he changed his shingle to read: "Alfred Solomon, MD. Family Practice and Psychotherapy."

Dr. S. counseled under the theories of Dr. Edmund Bergler, whose beliefs were not too far a cry from Freud's theories of psychoanalysis. Dr. Bergler held that those of us who suffer do so because we derive a sense of enjoyment from it. As babies, he argues, we neurotics feel refused by our mothers because they can't possibly attend to our every need. As a result, we find comfort in the familiar experience of being rejected, and continue to seek out situations where we can keep our pity-party going.

I wouldn't say that I did not benefit at all from my therapy with Dr. S. There were many times when I walked into his office feeling weak and forlorn, only to leave with a renewed bounce in my step. I would say that it was not the ideal therapy for me. One very important thing I did learn is this: Life will constantly bring frustrating and potentially negative situations our way, and we always have a choice. We can complain and suffer our lives away, or we can smile and try to see the good in everything.

♥
Rocky Mountain High

My good friend Keira was working in Calgary in the fall of my Year On. I saw visiting her as an excuse to see a new place and get away for a little while. When Keira had a few days off, we rented a car and set out to explore the Rocky Mountains near Lake Louise.

The first time we saw the mountains was at night. It was dark, but we could faintly make out their shapes – shadowy monsters whose awesome presence was impossible to ignore. When we saw them by day, particularly the Lake Louise vista, I was transformed.

I loved the mountains so much that after our three-day trip, I dropped Keira back in Calgary and drove up to Jasper via the Columbia Icefields Parkway. The drive from Lake Louise to Jasper on this road is easily one of the most picturesque 200 km stretches of road in the world.

Oct. 28/98

WOW – was I right about 'can't wait to get to the mountains'. This has by far been the highlight of my trip – if not my life. The Rockies are INCREDIBLE – beyond INCREDIBLE – <u>INDESCRIBABLE</u>! They are <u>so</u> beautiful – true beauty – and all so different. It made me think that art imitates all the patterns in nature – but of course can't come close because this stuff is <u>out</u> <u>of</u> <u>this</u> <u>world</u>! INCREDIBLE! AMAZING!

The entire time I was driving up and down the Icefields Parkway, I was beside-myself-overwhelmed with the majesty and beauty of these mountains. I had never seen anything like them before in my entire life. They made me feel small and they made God feel very large. I felt like I could have been swallowed up in a second by these beasts of nature, without anyone even noticing I was gone. I was humbled by the smallness of being a human being. I was praising the God that made this beautiful and awesome place on earth.

When I returned to Lake Louise for the second time that week, I went to the lake alone early in the morning. I walked along the periphery of the lake and stopped by a trickling waterfall. It was as if God was talking to me through the beauty of the waterfall. "What's your hurry to settle down?" God asked. "You're still young. Don't be in such a hurry."

I was puzzled by this message. I had been so ecstatic to finally find a soul-mate to share my life with, and now I was supposed to back off? I think God was telling me to take it easy, slow down, and be sure that I did the things that Bonnie needed to do before she settled down.

Lake Louise continues to be a place where I find it easy to connect with my spirit, and with God. I think the majesty of the natural world puts you closer to God, and closer to your soul's voice. The soul questions I was exploring at that time in my life pushed me to return to Lake Louise twice again within the next four years.

♥
Baltimore

On the night Nick and I got together, we both knew

that we would be partners for life. Details of wedding and marriage were only a matter of when and where.

I had only been working part-time in the fall of 1998, trying to get back on my feet after the attack of the *mystery illness*. In November, I drove with my family to Harrisburg, Pennsylvania to celebrate the American Thanksgiving with my cousins. Two days after Thanksgiving, we planned to pile into the family van to visit the National Aquarium. I told Nick over the phone about our plan and he joked that he would surprise me by showing up at the dolphin exhibit at noon. I warned him that these kinds of surprises require some planning.

It is interesting to hear the story from our two different perspectives. A melding of the two is equally amusing. After our casual conversation about meeting by the dolphins, Nick's boss received an email about special weekend fares on American Airlines. Baltimore was among the list of featured destinations. Nick had just picked up my engagement ring from the jeweler that day, and figured rather than risk losing it, he'd propose right away.

At my cousins, I was soon witness to a mysterious phone call. My younger cousin had handed the phone off to her mother, who proceeded to bolt upstairs with a look of confusion and urgency. Nick's plans were underway, and my cousin was now chief accomplice.

On Saturday November 28, 1998, Nick boarded a plane for Baltimore with a diamond ring burning a hole in his pocket. All seemed to be going according to plan.

Meanwhile, the happy tourists had left for Baltimore without incident. Upon arriving at the Aquarium, we found out that we were not allowed to enter until a designated time, for crowd-control reasons. We ate our packed lunches outside and enjoyed the unusually balmy November day in the attractive Baltimore harbor.

About half-way into his flight, Nick heard the announcement that every traveler dreads. The plane was going to be turned back to Toronto due to technical difficulties.

As we stepped off the entry escalator into the aquarium, my mother and cousin swiftly hustled us to the dolphin exhibit – a sure tip-off that Nick's plans were underway. Oddly though, Nick was nowhere to be seen.

Cleverly and inconspicuously, my mother left a note for Nick with the information booth explaining that we would return at 2:30 for the dolphin show.

Nick's plane finally arrived in Baltimore. Already late, he jumped into a cab and headed for the Aquarium.

We arrived at the dolphin show at 2:30, and Nick was still nowhere to be seen. Quickly taking stock of the large TV screens on either side of the pool, I had visions of being publicly embarrassed, of Nick (a non-swimmer) riding a dolphin with the ring between his teeth, TV screens announcing: **"BONNIE, WILL YOU MARRY ME?!"**

Thankfully, it was nothing like that. Nick arrived at the Aquarium in a near panic, and sweet-talked his way around the delayed entry policy. He rushed to the dolphin exhibit, only to find that his beloved and family were nowhere to be seen. He approached the information desk and asked if we could be paged. They refused. He tried another desk, where he explained his unique predicament. Finally, one woman said, "Are you Nick?" and handed him my mother's note.

I sat with my family waiting for the dolphin show to

begin, when I suddenly heard over my left shoulder: "Is this seat taken?" Half surprised and highly nervous, I belted Nick in the stomach. Not a great greeting for a guy that nearly killed himself to get there!

Nick joined us for the rest of the afternoon in the Aquarium. He insisted on lugging his winter jacket and overnight bag everywhere we went. The couple of times I suggested we get a locker for his belongings, he adamantly refused.

When we exited the aquarium, Nick pulled me aside to a bench in the harbor. He pulled out the ring, nervously proclaimed his abiding love for me, and I accepted his proposal. The rest, as they say, is history.

♥

Symptoms

All the while I was journeying off to the Rocky Mountains, being proposed to and working part-time, I was suffering from what I see now as typical anxiety symptoms: shortness of breath, heart palpitations, dizziness, a heavy feeling on my chest, and overwhelming fatigue. It seemed as though these symptoms would come and go when *they* pleased, which made my life feel very unpredictable. I was very frustrated because I felt like I didn't have control over my own health. Every time I made plans with someone, I was fearful that I wouldn't be able to fulfill them.

It did not occur to me for a long while that these symptoms could mean that I had anxiety or panic disorder. True, what I was experiencing looked a lot like something I had read on a website about anxiety, but no professional absolutely confirmed what I suspected. When I shared my suspicion with my family doctor, instead of diagnosing me, she sent me home with a pamphlet on anxiety. I eyed the checklist on the second page of the brochure, and it resembled what was going on with me. The information pamphlet was sponsored by a drug company, and the suggested treatment was medication. This was not a road I wanted to go down, so I didn't pursue it with my doctor.

I remember once asking my herbalist, who I saw much more often than my family physician, if my problem could be anxiety. His reply was: "It doesn't exist! There's no such thing as anxiety." Anxiety didn't fit into his model of diagnosing and healing.

Soon, the mystery illness was causing another problem: depression. It was a case of learned helplessness. Because of my perceived lack of control over my physical wellness, I was sad. In *The Anxiety and Phobia Workbook,* Edmund Bourne writes that, "Depression arises from feeling the grip of a condition over which you have no control or that you are powerless to change."[7] This is a perfect description of how I was feeling. Every time my symptoms returned, I would eventually slip into an end-of-the-world sob, singing the 'Why Me?' chorus long into the night.

Fortunately, though, I sought to find meaning in everything. During the 'Year On', my major was *me*. I asked. I probed. I tried on. I was not satisfied until *everything* made sense. Most of the time it did not, but some of the time it did. Fortunately, I asked a lot of the right questions: Was I happy? What did I want? Who was I? How could I get better?

---

[7]*The Anxiety and Phobia Workbook: Third Edition.* Edmund J. Bourne. (2000). Oakland, CA: New Harbinger Publications.

Panic

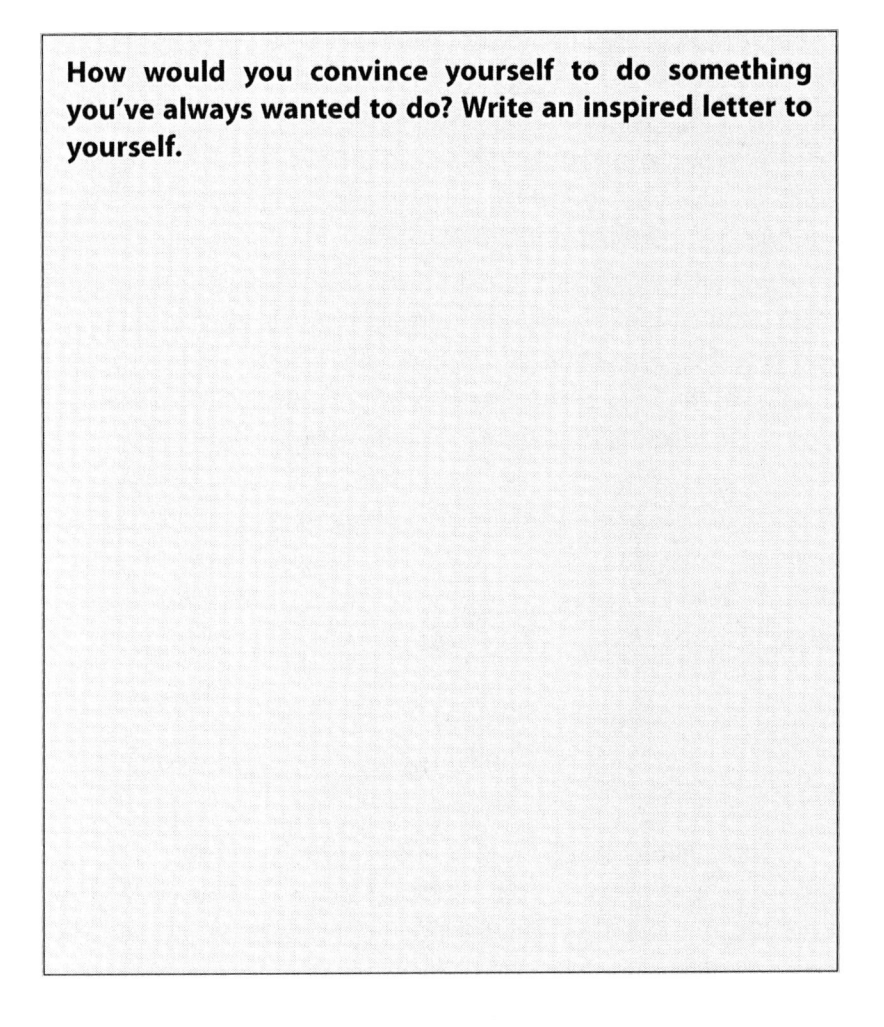

> **How would you convince yourself to do something you've always wanted to do? Write an inspired letter to yourself.**

Dec 6 /98

Bon,

This is a letter to you. Life is always going to bring you a challenge, and this will call on your strength (which you have, you just have to remember where it is). You have every right to be happy. Stop thinking you owe ANYONE ANYTHING. You don't. You owe only yourself. NO ONE is going to quit your job for you. You owe it to yourself. No one is going to plan your IDEAL trip. You owe it to yourself. You owe it to yourself to stop the world and find <u>YOUR</u> PLACE IN IT. Not the place you're <u>offered</u>, but the place YOU'VE FOUND. And if that means watching TV for A WEEK, then DO it, and please, please, please DON'T FEEL BAD ABOUT IT – <u>PLEASE!</u> (Because I think that's what you need to do!) And please don't worry about money (haven't we talked about this before?) Money is nothing. It's nothing, okay? (So maybe you should listen to Nick when he says his $ is our money.) Because it is. Because of what he told you last night. His $40,500 is nothing compared to the things you realize every day (and teach him) when you're living your life for you. You are a really smart person, and you have a lot more to teach yourself, and others. So go teach, and learn. You will feel like a valuable human being in this universe. LOVE, BON.

♥
Florida

When Nick bought my engagement ring, he was forced to postpone a trip to Southern California that he had been planning. Nick wanted to take me to Carlsbad, California where he had lived and worked for a year and a half. Instead, we went to stay at my parents' condominium in Florida for ten days.

When we first arrived, I promised myself that we would do this every year. The feeling of the sun beating down on my winter-frozen face was paradise four times over. It was so therapeutic.

Jan. 11, 1999
Here we are sitting on a beach in Marco Island, Florida, and I almost didn't know what day it was. Pretty

soon, I hope NOT to know what day it is. We came 2 days ago and it was HOT – that was exactly what I needed. Something totally fucking different from the Toronto grind we've been in. Especially since I wasn't feeling well in T.O. It's like suddenly I'm on vacation and a) I can't be sick b) I don't want to be and c) there's no reason to be because everything is so new, sunny, palm-treeing EXCITING! Which is perspective on the ENTIRE situation. Maybe I just need a <u>change</u> – a new perspective – a new city – a new climate – WHO KNOWS. All I know is that when we got to Thrifty rent-a-car in Ft. Lauderdale and the temperature was 80-something and I was <u>sweating</u> being OUTSIDE, I was REALLY happy. It dawned on me how important <u>change</u> is – to get the hell out of wherever you are and see something completely different JUST WHEN you think you're about to explode. Because there's more to life than your city, your house, your street and your job. There's OTHER STUFF – it doesn't matter what it is, it's just OTHER stuff and it gives you perspective on your life. There's not much perspective to be had when you're sitting in the shit. It's just shit all over.

♥
The Life You Were Born to Live

The joy I felt while in Florida gave me hope that heat and sun could heal my condition. It wasn't the first (or last) time I felt the 'this could be it!' feeling. I was yet to realize that there was no 'miracle cure'. Later, I would see that hard work and determination put into the right channels were the keys to overcoming panic disorder and anxiety.

While in Marco Island, Nick and I booked a 2-day

getaway to Disney World. Nick had never been to Disney and I couldn't wait to show him all the neat things about it.

The evening before we left on our getaway, I felt my symptoms returning. I felt the gnawing fatigue and loss of control over the events related to my health. I pulled out a book that had helped me many times before.

The Life You Were Born to Live by Dan Millman is a fantastic self-help book that is based on numerology. By adding the digits in your birth date you come up with your birth number, which in my case is 30/3. Here is how I get my birth number: November 17, 1973 is 1+1 (November is the 11th month) + 1 + 7 (my birth date) + 1 + 9 + 7 + 3 (my year of birth) = 30. The second '3' in 30/3 comes from adding the 3 and the 0 in 30 (3 + 0 = 3). The book contains several interesting sections, one of which describes each birth number in detail. This section contains specific information about your mission in life, your specific talents and the challenges you will be faced with. Dan Millman suggests that often what we are here on earth to do is what comes hardest to us.

Dan's insights are amazingly accurate. In my case, expression and sensitivity are my specific gifts. People born with my birth number make the best manic-depressives. We have a tendency to swing from incredible highs to the lowest lows. The key, he suggests, is to see each challenge as a hurdle to overcome, rather than a reason to stop trying and feel defeated.

In the back of Dan's book, you can read about specific laws that govern your birth number, such as "The Law of Honesty," "The Law of Faith" and "The Law of Action". This section contains other important details

Panic

about how to overcome a particular challenge you are facing.

Dan suggests that each year of your life also has a number attached to it, from 1 to 9. Each year in this cycle has characteristics associated with it. The year I was in Florida was a year 1 in my cycle, which corresponds with "newness, opening to new opportunities with confidence, planning and planting, resolutions and map-making."[8] This analysis was extremely accurate because it was the year I moved out of my parents' home.

Luckily, I had taken *The Life You Were Born To Live* with me on the trip to Florida. I read my life number again, I read the Laws in the back of the book that Dan had recommended, and it felt like a case of the right information at the right time. I was so motivated by what I read that it turned my mood right around. Dan asked me to think about "choosing to expand or contract; build or destroy in the area of creativity and expression." I thought about the things I *really* wanted, not just the things I was offered or fell into. I thought a lot about traveling. I thought about quitting my 'in-the-meantime' job. I made a list of things that I wanted to do with my life:

Jan. 19/99

• <u>TRAVEL</u> – *plan a trip for the spring /summer*

• *Talk to people about my experiences, thoughts and feelings*

• *Get married and on with my life and have kids and love them TO PIECES!!*

• *Maybe teach but somehow move people to be happier!*

---

[8] *The Life You Were Born To Live.* Dan Millman. (1993). Tiburon, CA: HJ Kramer.

I made a schedule of what I wanted the rest of my Year ON to look like. I brainstormed places to travel, I read and re-read my section in *The Life You Were Born To Live*.

I read the Law of Choices, which emphasizes that creative energy exists and must be channeled in positive ways or it will turn back on you and become destructive. This sounded like the reason I was sick. I realized that I hadn't spent nearly enough time asking myself what I wanted from my life. I needed my own place. I needed to travel. I needed to start a family.

Jan 19/99

Don't be a <u>VICTIM</u>. No <u>POOR ME</u>. Read something – do SOMETHING TO INSPIRE <u>YOU</u>. I will not be a victim. I will let my creative energy out positively.
KEEP THE VISION
TRIPS/TALKING/KIDS
What makes you tick – GO FOR IT! Or else you'll get sick again!

I continued to write in my journal when I came back from my trip:

Jan 25/99

Make a <u>CHANGE</u>
That's what Florida did for you – a CHANGE (in the direction of self-fulfilment) will pull you out of your darkness – something to let your creative genius free. Something you <u>LOVE</u> to do.

> **Being creative doesn't necessarily mean creating a piece of art or poetry. When we follow our hearts and share our unique gifts with the world, we are creating. How do you express your creative energy? How would you like to improve the ways that you express yourself?**

♥
How to Get What You Want and Want What You Have

In February of 1999, a month after the trip to Florida, I made an impulse buy at a bookstore. John Gray's *How to Get What You Want and Want What You Have:*

Bon's Year On

A Practical and Spiritual Guide to Personal Success jumped out at me in the bookstore and I couldn't put it down. I knew I needed to have the book, regardless of the hardcover price. Upon reading the first page, I saw that the book was dedicated to his wife, Bonnie. I took it as a sign.

How to Get What You Want is a remarkable book with many insights on life, love, personal needs, and how to satisfy them in the best way possible.

When reading John's book, I once again asked myself what I wanted from my life. In order to get what I wanted, I figured I'd need a clear picture of what that was. I continued to write my list of 'wants':

Feb. 22/99

<u>What do I want</u>?
1) To have time for <u>me</u>
- to reconnect with myself and my desires/needs
2) To see friends and do stuff
- shopping
- skating
- chatting
3) To travel for <u>ME</u> (maybe even alone)

Another part of Gray's book that was helpful was a small section on meditation. He suggests that meditation helps you to feel more connected to a higher power. Gray suggests you find a quiet place to sit and "with eyes closed, reach your hands up in the air a little above shoulder height or wherever is comfortable and begin repeating this phrase: 'Oh God, my heart is open to you, please come sit in my heart.'"[9] Gray suggests you

---
[9] *How to Get What You Want and Want What You Have: A Practical and Spiritual Guide to Personal Success.* John Gray. (1999). New York: HarperCollins.

repeat this phrase inside your head for about fifteen minutes. It is such a simple but powerful prayer.

I practiced this meditation. I did it at home. I did it while walking. I felt my fingers tingle while I welcomed God into my heart. I started to feel like I had more hope for my life because I was welcoming a higher power. I felt as though I was connected to a higher purpose. I felt that I was being cared for. Like Dan Millman, John Gray became another one of my teachers. It reminds me of the saying, "When the student is ready, the teacher will come".

What are some needs or wants that you have that would make you feel spiritually fuller?

Bon's Year On

♥
Automatic Writing

My friend Sam once told me about an excellent psychic he had gone to for a reading. Among other things, the psychic told him that he could communicate with his Spirit Guides through something called *automatic writing*. Spirit Guides are spirit entities that help you move along your spiritual path. Automatic writing gives you the opportunity to communicate to spirit guides by asking questions about your life. To prepare for automatic writing, Sam told me to create two columns on a piece of paper. Using cursive writing, Sam told me to pose a question for my spirit guides in the left column. Then I was to move to the right column, shift the pen to my non-dominant hand and "receive" the answer. This was where the automatic part of the writing was supposed to take over, just allowing the pen to move as it wanted to. And it did! At first, the writing that emerged was messy and illegible. After I practiced for a while, I got the hang of it. Some really interesting things came out. Here is a sample:

March 23/99
"*Hello Guardian Angel. Anything to say today?*"
Hold freedom.
Freedom is practice.
Feel free – Slow down.
Look out for the fast free.
Slow down from faster free.
You feel free fun.
Let yourself feel free.
You can do it.
Let down your freedom please.

Let Bonnie rest for once.
Keep up your friendships please.
You will feel free from them.
Press meetings for them.

Please understand that you are special for you understand some things within our world.

Understand that you can overcome anything by realizing that you could understand yourself and could lift from your pressures for understanding yourself is freedom from yourself.

Under under under under under under under under under under under could be your lock to past.

Under under your lock to the truth.

Freedom comes from unlocking the past from the present.

Please free the past from your present.

Please let my being free by understanding yourself from under the right place and do not ever doubt yourself. Because you can overcome everything if you are loving to yourself. Please do not ever love no something less than everyone because you are very very old.

Go think about your pressure. Do what you feel. Let out your fun. Please fun.

Wow! I thought that was so cool. Did all those words come from me? No, they came from the world of Spirit. The words were so poetic; so guiding; so urging; so wise. I loved the metaphor about "freeing the past from the present." It was as though my Higher Self was reminding me that I could be free from harmful patterns I had accumulated throughout my life. Three years later, when I found cognitive behavioral therapy, this wish would come true.

Bon's Year On

♥
Psychic Reading

While I have not been to many psychics in my lifetime, Doug Saunders[10] is by far the best one I've ever seen. My friend Sam highly recommended him, citing celebrity and police work among his credentials. I decided to give it a try.

My friend Jen and I were always interested in psychics, joking that we were "psychic sisters" in high school. I went to my appointment with Doug with an open mind, and got much more than I had anticipated. Interestingly, in a future reading, Doug told me that Jen and I *were* sisters in a former lifetime!

Doug's wife Jean, who books his appointments, told me to bring four personal items to the reading, such as a belt, hair brush, earrings, necklaces, rings or bracelets. Doug would hold on to these items during the reading to help him.

The reading was one of those things that felt right from the start. The condominium complex where Doug lives is nestled in a wooded area, and as I waited in his sitting room gazing out the window, two cardinals flew into my line of sight and rested on a branch. Those cardinals seemed to be looking at me and trying to tell me something. I have never forgotten that interesting moment. It made me feel that I was at the right place at the right time.

Jean called me into Doug's study and she asked me not to cross my legs or arms during the reading. She assured me that it was perfectly normal to feel warmth or chills during the session. I was allowed to take notes, but the session would not be audio taped.

---
[10] not his real name

Doug entered the room and shook my hand. He began by measuring the difference in length between my index and middle fingers. This indicated my ability to send and/or receive messages psychically. Doug said I am able to send and receive psychic material. Then he began with the reading. I wrote down everything he said, including the fact that I would write this book. I couldn't believe what I was hearing. I had never thought of writing a book. Doug went on to describe other amazing life events, as well as those of my future children.

When I asked him about my health problem, he told me that I was not really sick. He told me that I worry about dying young, but I won't. I would have a long life. He told me that I had a psychosomatic illness, and that I was a big worry wart. This couldn't have been more accurate. He suggested that my mind was overactive and did me harm. This characteristic is consistent with cognitive behavioral theories of anxiety disorders.

When the session finally ended, I realized that I had not even shown Doug the pictures I brought of family and friends for him to read. The time had gone so quickly, but I was not disappointed. I left feeling giggly and excited. Not so much about the future books as the future children. I felt like I had actually met them. I could picture them in my mind's eye. Doug's reading had the ability to put me in touch with my future, if just for a moment, and that was powerful.

♥
First attempt at "The Book"

Feb. 20/99, 7am
When I was 24, I dropped out of graduate school

because it was making me miserable. This was the beginning of a chain of events that led me to better health. Health to me has become a multi-faceted word that includes much more than my physical well-being. The outcome is often PHYSICAL health, but the underlying process addresses all facets of my life – emotional, psychological, spiritual to name a few. I believe that physical health cannot be obtained until we recognize that we are very alive, three-dimensional organisms in a vastly complex world. It is naive to think that treating a physical symptom will lead to long-term health because most often this does not address the cause of an illness, which could be any number of things on any number of levels (emotional, psychological, spiritual, etc.).

This philosophy is what brought me to healing. I became an active participant in my healing when I began looking at various aspects of my life. I started asking myself if I was happy in my job. Was I happy as a person? Were there areas of my life that could use some improvement? My conclusion (which is an ever-changing, ever-evolving process) was that I had to quit my job, reconsider my plans to go to school in the fall (for my 7th year of university) and think more about how I respond to illness. My illness. For as soon as I stepped out of victim mode (poor me- why is this happening to such a good person, and for so <u>LONG</u>?), I empowered myself to become my own healer. This is not to say I didn't use others as resources. I certainly did. But the key to using other sources was that I knew my body (and mind) best (most of the time) and that I was the best judge of what was and wasn't good for me AT THAT TIME.

Knowing myself is easier said than done, especially when there are so many people who tell you to see a doctor who can give you a pill....

*My hope in writing a book is to reach others who have, or **are** undergoing a similar experience to mine. The common name is "psychosomatic illness" in the Western medical world, but I prefer to see it as a spiritual illness. There was an essential part of me that wasn't being heard, and so my body became sick to get me to listen up. You will listen to your body, but it is easy to ignore your mind. When your spirit cannot stand being ignored any more, it will use your body as a messenger.*

It is my hope that someone, even one person, will look at their illness and say: "I can overcome this". It is my hope that they will see themselves as a three-dimensional human being, with wants, needs and desires that cannot be satisfied simply by popping a few pills. It is my hope that that same person can have the courage to look at their life and see where there may be some improvements made.

I believe that we are here on earth to be the best that we can be. Unfortunately, there are many hurdles to becoming a healthy, vibrant human being in our society. There are so many blatant and hidden messages in our society that prevent fulfillment from being our main purpose in life. Our society tells us to make money, and perhaps the things you attain with that money will make you happy. This could not be further from the truth. Right now, I have 45 dollars in my bank account. I am living in my parents' house, but I am happy because I feel fulfilled writing these words....

My hope is that, despite all of society's messages that argue otherwise, someone will say: I believe in myself. I can be in control of my life and my healing. I know myself best. I will make it my mission to know myself even better, and to take those necessary steps towards better health. Better spiritual health. There is no other way.

Do you have a manifesto? What do you strongly believe?

Panic

Feb. 20, 1999

<u>Things that have helped me</u>

- Dan Millman's <u>The Life You Were Born to Live</u>
- Walking outdoors
- Doing what I feel like doing, when I feel like doing it.
- Journal writing
- The Rocky Mountains
- Talking with my ever-patient and loving fiancé, Nick
- My herbalist Diego
- Drawing
- Thinking
- Reading a bit from many books, when I needed them
- Realizing I'm a pretty funky person.
- SARK's <u>Bodacious Book Of Succulence</u>
- Dr. Alfred Solomon and Berglerian therapy
- Learning it's o.k. to watch tv sometimes
- REIKI and the wisdom of Denise Crundall
- Reading Gary Zukav's <u>The Seat of the Soul</u>
- Accidentally fumbling upon Oprah's show when she has wonderfully spiritual guests such as Gary Zukav and John Gray
- Listening to music i.e. Sheryl Crow's Every Day is a Winding Road
- The movie What Dreams May Come
- Dancing around my room with the music turned up really loud
- A funeral
- Talking with my friend Keira, a wonderfully intelligent and grounded human being
- Planning a wedding and growing up
- People who were willing to listen
- Most importantly:
  ME! because I chose to do all these things

Make a list of people, experiences or things that have helped you become more spiritually, emotionally, mentally or physically healthy.

♥
The Apartment

After my first year of university, I moved back home to continue my studies in Toronto. I had not saved appropriately for four years of living away, and couldn't stand to be away from Stephen, so this made good sense.

Once I finished my undergraduate degree and started my Master's, I again felt a strong need to leave home. At 23, I was hoping that Stephen and I could find a small, inexpensive apartment on campus. My initial investigation revealed that the cheapest apartments were an astounding $700 a month. My graduate student salary of $1000 per month made this an unlikely option. Moving out was not meant to happen at that time.

Fast forward two years to 'The Year On'. I was in a completely different head space, yet with the same need of having a space of my own. I started looking again for apartments in safe neighborhoods, jotting down phone numbers and inquiring about rental costs.

During this time, I placed a call to a friend whose father owned an apartment building in one of the neighborhoods I liked. I told him that Nick and I would be looking to move in after our wedding in December. He ended up calling us much sooner than I expected, and asked if I would be interested in a one-bedroom beginning May 1st.

Wow! Eight months before we needed a place. Eight months before *we* needed a place. I wrestled with the idea of moving in so soon before the wedding and it began to grow on me...

Mar 1/99

Dear Nick,

I am writing something to you that will at the same time be difficult, but is also a relief to hear.

As I asked for guidance in the matter of this apartment, something became clear to me.

<u>We</u> are not the ones that need this apartment. <u>I</u> am.

<u>We</u> are not the ones that can't wait to move out. <u>I</u> am.

And therefore, <u>WE</u> should not be the ones to take this apartment. <u>I</u> should.

It seems totally impractical – but that's not why I need to do this. LOGIC, for ONCE IN MY LIFE, plays NO PART IN THIS. It doesn't make sense for <u>us</u>, because it's supposed to happen for <u>ME</u>.

I'm the one who needs this, and so I'm the one who will take responsibility for this. I can't have you feeling responsible for my shit. Husband or not, I will always be <u>ME</u>, and you will always be you.

So right now, Bonnie <u>NEEDS</u> her own space. And for once, Bonnie is going to make sure that's what Bonnie gets. I really owe it to myself Nicky. I really do. I want this so badly I can't tell you. Please try to understand. It is such a relief to write this that I have tears in my eyes. Not telling <u>you</u> what I need, but telling <u>MYSELF</u>. Allowing myself to <u>need</u>. Allowing logic to go to the wind for <u>ONCE</u>. I'm going to spoil ME for once no matter what it takes. Because <u>I deserve it</u>...

I CAN DO THIS, and all I need is your support. Emotional, not financial. I just need (or want) you to say: "Bon, I can see why you need to do this. Financially it is not feasible for me now...I love you and I will do my best to support you in this"....

I love you. And I trust me. Please be there for me now.

I need you to believe in me. Yours forever with lots and lots of love, Bon XO

I moved in May 1st.

> **Write a letter to your partner communicating something that is difficult to say out loud. If you don't have a partner, write a letter to an important person in your life that you would like to communicate with on a deeper level.**

Bon's Year On

♥
The Two-Headed Monster

While the apartment was a wonderful step in the right direction, it brought out an all-new two-headed monster in perfectionism. In my therapy with Dr. Solomon, I had come to understand that my high-achieving perfectionist tendencies had the power to get me in quite a bit of psychological trouble. Suffering, both physical and mental, occurred as a result of the real world not living up to my imagined ideal of how it was supposed to be.

Transition is never a good time for a perfectionist. Boxes all over, dirty floors, people sitting on misplaced chairs, it was a mental disaster waiting to happen. In fact, well before the move to the apartment, I started to feel the physical symptoms return. Exhaustion, heart palpitations and dizziness were par for the course.

Moving day. I had accrued a superb team of male strength: my father, my (future) father-in-law, my friend Sam, my (future) brother-in-law Joe, my brother Rafi, Nick, and Nick's friend Vito. It was a beautiful May morning, the heat of summer threatening to arrive prematurely.

Nick and his brother picked up the cube van on schedule, making their first stop at my grandparents' to pick up my bed. By the time they arrived at my house, I was feeling so weak that I couldn't lift a thing.

I was the foreman, if a slightly embarrassed mentally shrinking woman could be called that. I politely asked my friend Sam, who was, aside from Nick, the only one in on my condition, to retrieve bags and boxes from my room upstairs. I was glad to have the help, but embarrassed to be the way I was. It was the familiar *not-being-able-to-explain-to-people-who-only-understand-physical-disorders* problem, which only added to the stress of the day. I knew that I was sick, unwell, compromised in some way, but I didn't have a label for it yet. And even if I did, I sure wasn't going to go around advertising that I, a perfectly capable woman in her 20s who graduated Magna Cum Laude from university, *had a mental disorder!* Are you crazy?

The first few days in the apartment were tumultuous for my head and body. To an outsider, the place probably just looked like a normal apartment in the middle of a move. I needed things to be just-so, right away. Dealing with the time between here and perfect was torture. I didn't understand why it took *time* to make the apartment look as I had envisioned it. Patience was a virtue hard to come by.

♥
Space

I was definitely right about one thing: I *needed* that apartment. For all the reasons I suspected, the first being distance from my parents' home. Not necessarily a far distance, I just needed to be in a different space. It was time to live with me, in me, surrounded by me.

Once I was living there for a little while, I started to notice things dropping off. Patterns, habits, and ways of doing things that I discovered were not even mine to begin with. They were my mother's, or my father's, or my grandparents', but they were not mine. I was becoming someone else, but really just more myself. It felt really good to be able to figure out where *I* was under those things that weren't mine.

Bon's Year On

♥
Inspiration

July 24, 1999

I've just got to say this – it's Sat. morning, and I'm just sitting in the apartment and listening to music, and writing in the big chair by the window, and I'm palpitating BUT I'M SO HAPPY TO BE IN THE MOMENT – <u>this</u> moment of calm (hope that made sense, because it really does feel like a breakthrough, not to feel an urgency that I have to GO SOMEWHERE or whatever. Yahoo!)

Something has shifted.

The job of the human race is not to feel guilt about NOT being something. It is simply to be EXACTLY where you are. Which is not the easiest thing, considering how often we're told where to be, what to eat, and how to think. Let's try to teach BE YOU. How about you (and you, and you) are on a sacred path which is so incredibly beautiful because it is <u>YOURS</u>! And the best thing you can do in this life is to step up to the plate and take a swing. AT YOUR LIFE. Be the best you can be, despite what the WHOLE ENTIRE WORLD SAYS. You are the big boss of yourself. You have been given that gift. Use it with the care you would give the most precious gift in the world. God gave us the gift of free will, and too many people abuse it. Once you discover that it is a GIFT, try not to treat it as if it is a RIGHT.

I find it tough to claim that gift. Because I have internalized so many expectations. And I'm also very afraid to go against the grain and ROCK THE BOAT. Afraid people will be MAD AT ME – ooooh – wouldn't that be HORRIBLE...

IT'S <u>MY</u> LIFE. And I don't think I've ever REALLY

TRULY felt like it was. It was always mine and someone else's.

IT'S MY LIFE. IT'S MY LIFE. (This is making me cry realizing that.) WOW!

IT'S MY LIFE. IT'S TOTALLY MY LIFE. IT'S MY LIFE. IT'S MY LIFE. OH MY GOD WHAT WILL I DO WITH IT. I FEEL LIKE I'VE JUST BEEN GIVEN A GIFT THAT I DON'T KNOW WHAT TO DO WITH. OH MY GOD ALL OF A SUDDEN I REALIZE I HAVE TOTAL RESPONSIBILITY.

WOW! I NEVER EVER EVER REALIZED IT WAS TOTALLY, COMPLETELY 100% MINE. It's the gift I just wrote about. WOW. Scary.

Maybe this whole thing has been a process of RE-CLAIMING. No longer FALLING INTO, but consciously acting. Which, as far as I can tell, has purely and simply come from hard work, perseverance and the grace of God.

How would your life be different if you didn't think so much about other people's expectations of you? What kind of positive change could you make in your life if you only thought of yourself?

♥
The Cottage

In the summer of 1999, my very best friend Jen decided I needed a little 'cottage healing'. Her parents had rented a cottage a couple of hours northeast of the city, and Jen thought it would be a great idea if we escaped for five days of R&R. A completely generous suggestion.

Jenny Clarke and I met in Junior High School, and it didn't take long before we were inseparable. We spent many summers, falls, springs and winters together. We skied, studied, and became camp counselors together. On summer weekends in between camp sessions, we would escape to her family's cottage and hang out. This was about as good as life gets. Swimming, boating, throwing the Frisbee, playing cheesy arcade games, eating, and sleeping. No responsibilities other than applying enough sunscreen and being pleasant and helpful to Jen's mom and dad, which was easy.

So when Jen suggested we join her parents at the cottage, it seemed like a throw-back to old times. I didn't say no, but I was worried about how I would feel. I once bought a greeting card by Mary Engelbreit that says: *"Worrying does not empty tomorrow of its troubles. It empties today of its strength."* That couldn't have been more true the morning Jen was supposed to pick me up for the trip to the cottage. I was so nervous, and then my heart started palpitating, so much so that I begged Nick not to make me go. I couldn't even cry because then the palpitating got worse.

Jen arrived, and I got my things together. We drove off and thus began Palpitation Week. I palpitated in my sleep, I palpitated when I ate, I palpitated when I paddled, and it drove me nuts! I really got upset. The "Why Me?" feeling was all-too familiar. I was in tears one evening when Jen asked if I wanted to run to the corner store with her and her parents. "I just don't feel well," I sniffled, and my heart broke. Why couldn't I just be normal again? What the HELL was the matter with me?

The one thing that did make me feel calm that week was Jen's dad. He has such a laid-back attitude towards life, and his voice is very soothing. One evening when we all went out for dinner, I enjoyed listening to him talk because it made me feel like everything was going to be okay.

Ironically, as soon as Jen and I pulled out of the cottage driveway to go home, my heart palpitations suddenly stopped. "Gimme a break," I thought. "Now I want to go back!" In retrospect, though, the timing made perfect sense.

I soon learned the technical name for the cause of my suffering at the cottage. "Anticipatory anxiety" is a feeling of anxiety over a future event. There may or may not be just cause for this anxiousness, usually not. I felt anxious before leaving for the cottage because I was anticipating that I would feel bad when I got there. I would be away from the comforts of my home, and away from Nick. What if I had a panic attack? Who would understand? Who would comfort me?

Actually, I didn't really go so far as to put a face on the predicted disasters ahead. I worried vaguely. With my cognitive behavioural therapist, I later learned to paint a detailed picture of my fears. Only then could I see that the anticipated "big scary thing" was seldom as big and scary as I thought.

Reflect on common worries you have that never seem to come true. Make a list of these worries as a reminder that they're not worth your time and energy.

♥
Cold Feet

Worry about my wedding day started well before December of 1999. In July of that year, I debated postponing the wedding because of my unpredictable state of health. Why not wait until I was better, I reasoned. It didn't seem smart to plan for a wedding that I may or may not be able to enjoy.

When I confessed this idea to my mother, she thought I might be experiencing the common "cold feet" phenomenon. Mothers are always right, though we're never willing to admit it at the time.

July 23/99

…I started freaking out about the implications of being married for BONNIE, who loves Nick dearly, but still feels she hasn't fulfilled herself as an independent woman. I really need to consider a lot of things and take stock.

I've spent my life doing what I thought I wanted, and what I thought others wanted was more what happened.

What's funny is that when I went out west in the fall, the one thing that occurred to me (hear God on the whisper?) is that I'm in too much of a hurry – that I've got a lot of life to live.

And it really truly freaks the hell out of me that I could not be able to <u>stand</u> through my marriage ceremony.

IRONIC, though, that I have to get sick (AGAIN?!) to re-assess what I'm doing. Hmmm…

WHY IS THIS ALWAYS HAPPENING? …AND …NO! Stop the questions and guess work, and LIVE!!

<u>SO</u>, I look forward to the opportunity to reassess and to HEAL.

The wedding date did not change. Nick and I had a lot of talks about it. He decided he could not handle the change of date after we had already booked everything, not to mention having to try to explain the reasons to family and friends. I still knew I wanted to marry Nick, but I think I felt a little arm-wrestled into remaining true to the original plan. I would find my way, however, to assert my independence and womanhood by taking solo trips for the next couple of years, despite the fact that I was a married woman.

♥
Sam's Readings

When my friend Sam visited the psychic, he learned how to do psychic readings of his own, and I was glad to have him use me as his guinea pig. I was happy to be on the receiving end, especially once I realized how accurate he could be. Sam spoke in imagery when he began his readings. He once described me sitting in a boat, paddling towards a sunset past signs that read "slow down!" In his reading, he saw me saying: "To you it's just the sunset, but to me it's the sun," to which a voice replied: "The sun will always be there – no rush to go to it. If you go too fast you won't have time to enjoy it. Enjoy it."

Before one reading, Sam did some automatic writing from a spirit guide. What he wrote and handed to me was just amazing:

> *July 28/99*
> *...feel life Bonnie, feel love for your soul has not felt life once before. Oh Bonnie you got so much life and love to give. Be open to new experiences. You are doing well but must keep your faith in rough waters. You have been chosen to live a life of love and happiness. Peace Bonnie and be open but not vulnerable. Peace, friend, peace.*
>
> *Believe in yourself and do not separate your spirituality from your emotions. You need to keep your soul connected to you. When you are in another state of mind – in despair – then you lose your balance and power. Stay in control – you are the boss – not your sicknesses. You must keep your inner power when weakness takes over you physically. Bonnie when you are feeling not in control then you become vulnerable to your emotional state. When this happens then how can you be in control? Bonnie you will agree with me because I speak to you from love. You are special to my Sam so you must then be special to me. Fear not. Fear tricks your emotional state. Fear is not stronger than faith.*

FEAR IS NOT STRONGER THAN FAITH became my mantra for some time after that. I was so appreciative to Sam for taking the time to help me with his gift.

♥
OISE/UT

The Year On came to a close, and it was time to start teachers' college. The week before the start of classes, my heart started to beat funny again. There was no way I was going to let heart palpitations put off school for another year. So I borrowed Nick's car, swallowed the overpriced parking rates for one day, and braved the first day of class. Though I was feeling weak, I soon realized that I was at the right place at the right time. The professor that welcomed our group spoke in metaphors: We were now caterpillars that would cocoon ourselves and emerge as teacher-butterflies by spring. Margie Buttignol was sweet, sensitive, and exactly the kind of person I needed in my corner the year I emerged from my Year On. I did not hesitate to approach her at the end of the morning to ask for her understanding with regard to my "condition".

"Oh, you're just a sensitive person," she reassured me, and made mention of a book that she had recently read about the highly sensitive individual. I knew I was in the right hands.

That fall, I was sure I was anemic. After sitting in class for 6 ½ hours, I would usually rush straight home on the subway. I would soon be laid out on the couch for the rest of the evening. Weekends were the same, minus the 6 ½ hours in school. A simple blood test confirmed my anemia suspicion. However, the iron pills my doctor prescribed made me constipated, which is a common side effect, so I went on to try something else. Again.

In *Vitality,* Toronto's free monthly health magazine, I found the name of a highly qualified acupuncturist from China. I decided to try acupuncture, hoping again for a magic cure. The needles did hurt going in so I guess the acupuncturist wanted to get right at the root of the problem. Though the acupuncture provided some short-term relief, in the long term I still suffered from a variety of symptoms.

Then again, if the root of my problem was not physical, why should I have expected to feel better?

♥
My Big Fat Italian/Jewish Wedding

The year I was in teachers' college was also the year I got married – superb planning for a person with anxiety issues. Nick and I wanted to move in together, but our families' traditional views on co-habitating prevented us from spending more than weekends together in my apartment.

November, the month before the wedding, was also when I was doing my first teaching block. I was responsible for planning and teaching increasing amounts of curriculum, running around in the evenings with Nick to our last-minute wedding appointments, and dealing with the fact that my grandmother was going under the knife for colon cancer. It would have been an extremely stressful time for anyone, but for a person with anxiety it was a recipe for disaster.

I was extremely stressed and hadn't yet established an effective method for managing it. I remember trusting in the power of sleep – that was my best strategy. Nights seemed to be the only time I had to myself, and I put faith in those seven or eight hours to give me the nourishment I so badly needed.

On the last day of my teaching placement, the inevitable happened. By early afternoon, I could literally feel the energy dripping from my body. That drained feeling was the perfect setup for a panic attack. To make things worse, I had been put in charge of the class because there was a substitute teacher for the day. Unfortunately, I was so panicked that I couldn't even get myself off the teacher's chair. I was happy to hide behind the desk trying desperately to disappear. The elderly substitute teacher was becoming increasingly frustrated that I was not fulfilling my duties. And to make matters worse, I couldn't assert my need to go home and rest.

Dec. 1/99

WOW! December already! It feels official now. 17 days. I really am praying. I started feeling badly last week, and managed to make my way to the end of the teaching block. But Saturday I woke up and felt horrible. Like every bit of energy was being drained from my body. Scary because my "stagette/shower" was that night. I spent a lot of the day fretting the party because I wanted to be okay. I went, and in the first half hour I thought I was going to pass out. But I didn't, and things got better. I was okay for most of it, but got a wicked headache near the end.

Write about a specific time or event that caused you to be overly anxious, but then didn't turn out as badly as you expected.

♥
Connie

My friend Sam's mother is a born-again Christian and often performs healing prayers on those who ask for her help. I once asked Sam if he thought she would mind me calling her, despite the fact that I was Jewish. He understood that I wasn't looking to be converted, just desperate for healing in any way, shape or form. Sam had mentioned me to his mother before, and said that she would definitely welcome the call.

The first time I called, I was a little nervous but Connie was so reassuring and gentle that I immediately felt the power of the healing she channeled from God. When I started speaking to her, it was as though a truth serum had been injected into my soul. All my fears and truths came pouring out, along with some tears which I tried to hide. Connie is such a loving, clear, and positive person.

When I called again just before my wedding, I explained that the big day was coming up in a couple of weeks and that I felt weak and afraid. Connie and I talked a bit first, and then she prayed for me. I paid close attention to the soothing words she spoke in our conversation and wrote some of them down in my journal to look back on.

Sam explained to me that images will often come into his mother's mind when she is praying for someone, and in my case, she had visualized a kind of depression.

Sam was in my wedding party, so his mother knew the exact date of the wedding. After the fact, he told me that she had prayed the entire day for us.

When you are in a state of great anxiety, what do you need to hear to calm your fears? What would you want an unconditionally loving person or being say to you to make you feel beter?

Panic

♥
Wedding Day and Guardian Angels

Dec. 23/99
What an amazing, amazing day. I can't believe it happened to me. And I can't believe it's over. Wow.
The alarm went off at 6 am, and Jen had slept over. As promised we had watched When Harry Met Sally the night before. But it was frequently interrupted with "I just thought of something," followed by a frantic rummaging through the bedroom closet, or bathroom medicine cabinet.
We had spent a long day searching for the perfect "over the wedding dress" jacket at Fairview Mall, including a run to Hallmark for my garter (which Jen later engineered to look perfectly beautiful) and an earlier trip to the salon for 2 French manicures. By the end of the day, my legs were aching, but I had that jacket, and it was great... fuzzy white and everything.
The 6 am alarm was followed by Jen's excited words: "Today's the day you're getting married!"

The memories that continued to pour from my pen weren't necessarily the typical wedding moments, like walking down the aisle, kissing at the altar, and dancing our first dance. Those moments were carefully recorded on video and in pictures. The moments that made their way into the pages of my journal were the odd in-between ones, like sitting at the hair-dresser in the morning, chatting with Sam in between the ceremonies, sitting in the limo with my friends thinking, "we should do this again some time!"

I didn't know that Connie had been praying for us

all day. But in retrospect, it makes sense because I had visions beyond the everyday at the reception.

During a Jewish wedding, there is always at least one hora, a circle dance where the bride and groom are lifted onto chairs in the middle of the circle while people dance around them. When the looks of terror on the bride and groom's faces indicate it's time to release them to the ground, they then join the Hora with everyone else. I was afraid that during the dance, my heart palpitations would surface. I was afraid that I would pass out. I was afraid that I would make a fool of myself. I was afraid that people would think I was weak, helpless, incapable. Then Howie came to mind.

When I was eleven, our very close family friend Howie died from a brain tumor. When I started having difficulty with my health, he started to come to mind. At the strangest times I would feel his presence, and it was undeniable. He was often there with me to help me through a rough patch.

On my wedding day, Howie was there again. When I expressed my fear about passing out, Howie answered. "If you fall, *I'll* catch you". That was that. I danced.

I also felt the presence of my maternal grandparents. My mother's mother passed away before I was born, and my grandfather had passed away just two-and-a-half years before the wedding. I really felt like they were there. Their presence was strong. Why wouldn't they have been? Their only daughter's daughter was getting married. I felt their blessing. More than that, in my mind's eye I could see them dancing. They were there on the dance floor with us, holding each other in a way they hadn't been able to since 1972, the year my grandmother died. I could sense that my grandfather was pleased to be with his wife. Then, after the last dance, they left. I saw them go. They waved goodbye and thanked me for the simcha.[11] It was amazing.

In my speech, I mentioned that I felt the presence of my maternal grandparents at the wedding. I'm not sure how many people believed me, but I hope my mother did. Her parents were proud.

♥
Honeymoon

Our honeymoon fell over the Millennium New Year, so we were careful to select a destination where we would not have to spend a fortune. For a reasonable price, we found an all-suite, five star property in Costa Rica.

Before we left, I was feeling tired. I'm not sure whether the wedding craziness had finally caught up with me, but the all-familiar drained feeling hit hard the night before we were supposed to leave. Friends that had come from Chicago for the wedding wanted to stop by, and even though I ordinarily would have loved to visit with them, on that night I really wanted to say no. I didn't feel I could handle it. I thought I was going to melt, faint, drop, *have a panic attack*, but I said yes because we see each other so infrequently.

I borrowed from empty and feigned conversation for a couple of hours. Once our friends left, I dropped. Nick had to finish off the packing, and we woke up at 4:30 am to catch our flight.

I'm glad we chose to go away for two weeks because the first week in Costa Rica was a mess. It didn't get off to a great start when our plane was detained in Panama

---
[11] Yiddish word for a milestone celebration (e.g., wedding, bar-mitzvah)

City for four hours. The only restaurant in the airport served at a Latin American pace, and I was starving. When we arrived in Costa Rica, we boarded a coach to take us to the resort. The roads in Costa Rica have enormous potholes due to the rains. After two hours of swerving, stopping and starting, we finally arrived, only to stand in line forever to check into the hotel.

Luckily, the resort was absolutely beautiful. The breakfasts were plentiful. And the company was wonderful. But I had trouble enjoying it because of my symptoms. I was drained and nauseous, and then I got the flu – fever and all. The first week of our honeymoon didn't feel much like a honeymoon and I guess that made me feel even worse.

I cried. Once again, I hit the wall of despair. Poor me. Why me? Why now? Desperate, I called Connie. I needed someone to pray for me and to help me pray right.

Yet again, Connie's soothing voice and prayer cheered me up. She told me to fight the drained feeling – to go out, swim, walk – to stop being a victim of these forces.

Her prayer and my determination became a powerful team. I fought the fatigue and got into the shower. Though I felt dragged down by some mysterious force, I struggled with all my might. I got dressed and we went for dinner. I was determined to take control.

The next couple of days we lounged by the spectacular pool and swam. We went for a couple of fancy dinners. We took a taxi into town and explored. We signed up for a day trip to an active volcano and we swam in natural hot springs. We finally started to enjoy our vacation. It was a victory quite unlike any other.

♥
Home Again

I returned to teachers' college after my honeymoon to open arms. In just four months, I had grown quite close to my classmates and professors. They were eager to hear all the details of my special day. My friend Susie, also a teacher, had warned me to take an extra day off after I came back from my honeymoon to get settled. "Don't rush right back in," she suggested. "Just do your laundry and take it easy." She was absolutely right, but I had missed two days of school already, and didn't want to miss the beginning of a new course on the third day. So I went.

Although my rush to return to class may not have ruined things altogether for second semester, my worrying and hyper-vigilance may have. About a month into the term, I got a run-of-the-mill fever. I also got that drained feeling again. I remember calling my professor, worried about missing classes.

"You just got *married*!" she said. "Of *course* you're tired. Take a couple of days, and don't rush back. You need to take it easy."

I was relieved that she was so understanding. In fact, I lucked out that year, because most of my professors were that understanding. I was blessed. I was worried.

My fever kept returning when I tried to go back to school or to my teaching placement, and I was also feeling dizzy. I made an appointment with my doctor who diagnosed an inner ear infection.

"It usually takes about six weeks to three months to recover," she said. "There is no treatment because it is a virus. You just have to wait it out."

I freaked out. Teachers' college did not allow students

to miss that much time if they wanted to graduate with the rest of their class, so being away three months was not an option. I went to my herbalist.

"Yes, it is an inner ear infection." Hallelujah, a consensus! "I'll do some energy healing and that should take care of it."

Fortunately, the energy healing did work and I felt better for a little while. But then the dizziness returned.

"You are being reinfected somewhere," my herbalist said. "Let me try to find out where."

I explained that I was practice teaching in a very old school downtown, and that whenever I went back, I got the fever again.

"Aha!" he said, after consulting with his spirit guides. "The washroom at the school is doing this to you. The germs are there. Don't use that washroom."

Okay, sure. I was so frustrated that I was willing to try anything.

Then I got sick *again*. Another trip to Diego.

"Hmmm. Let me see..." he paused, asking his guides questions in his head, while touching my ear and using his muscle tester.

"It's in your house. Somewhere in your house something is holding the infection, and reinfecting you." Okay, I thought. Then why isn't Nick getting sick? And all those people in the school. They're okay.

"The washroom! It's the washroom," he concluded. "Get a spray bottle, fill it with alcohol. Then hold the bottle for one minute and say this prayer. Then spray your entire washroom. Spray your sheets, too. Your bed might have the infection. And spray the clothes you wear."

In retrospect, I see how silly this seems. I was a believer, though. I didn't think to doubt, especially because I needed a miracle cure. Anxiety and panic as a cause for my illness were far from my mind. I bought the spray bottle. I went nuts. My whole apartment smelled like rubbing alcohol. It still took five weeks to get better.

I missed almost an entire teaching block which gave me more reason to worry. I was sick and I wasn't getting better, and there was a risk of not being able to graduate because of missed practice teaching days.

I called my professor again in a panic.

"You have an inner ear infection! Of course you need to rest. Please do not worry. You *will* graduate – I will make sure of that. You will make up your practice teaching days. Please don't worry and just concentrate on getting better."

Oh boy, easier said than done. A person with anxiety who has not had the right kind of therapy does not stop worrying. We twist and turn and writhe in pain, but we do not stop worrying. We know this is not in our best interest, but we do not stop worrying. We get sicker, but we do not stop worrying. We would love to stop worrying, but we do not know how.

I did recover from the inner ear infection, and fortunately, I was able to make up my practice teaching time. At the end of our program, we all had to participate in a month-long internship at a school of our choice. Thanks to a little administrative massaging by my wonderful professor, I made up the missed practice teaching time during the internship – in Sam's split grade one/two classroom, of all places. I thought that I would enjoy spending a month with Sam learning and playing.

Internship month was also interview month, when all the boards of education started calling the future graduates. Although we all knew the questions and the answers before we walked in, it was still nerve-wracking. My grandparents, whom I had been visiting at lunch hour because they lived across the street from Sam's school, could tell I was stressed. My appetite was non-existent and I was again playing host to a whole list of anxiety symptoms. Heart palpitations, debilitating fatigue, light-headedness. Sam was understanding, which I was lucky for, but sometimes, I just had to swallow whatever piece of suffering was taking place and teach.

Then there was the matter of the students. I couldn't believe how rude, disobedient, and frustrating children could be until I had that placement. I was questioning my career choice in the same week that I was running to interviews.

April 29/00

I don't know if this teaching thing is for me. When there's a tough class (like Sam's) it takes everything out of you and gives you nothing in return. Big megalomaniacs, those kids.

It's hard because you have to have control of the kids but it takes too much to control THESE kids. Then there's this health matter. Causes strife, because I have even LESS energy, and the kids drain me.

Oh no. HELP. I don't know what to do.

I made it through, and by June, I did graduate with the rest of my class. On graduation day, I felt mild anxiety symptoms. Was my heart beating funny? Did I have enough energy? Would I pass out in front of all those people? It was a constant drone in my mind. But of course, I crossed the stage without incident.

♥
Rocky Mountains, Part Two

Seeing the Rocky Mountains once was not enough for me. After I graduated from teachers' college, I set off on a second trip out West. This time, there was no friend to stay with, and only the open road as my companion. That didn't bother me. I couldn't wait to get back out to see my old friend, Lake Louise.

I booked the trip at the last minute. I remember trying to decide on the *perfect* day to go and the *perfect* day to come back. I didn't yet realize that sometimes, you just have to go with the best decision you know how to make at that time. Booking a flight became more of a melodrama than it needed to be, as with many more things in my life. I finally decided that I would leave the day after graduation. Ten days out west would be enough, and all I could afford. I would fly to Calgary, rent a car, drive to the Rockies, spend a couple of days there, and then drive west towards Vancouver, ending my trip in Whistler. WOW! What a great itinerary.

Yes, it was WOW! And then WOW again, and then some more WOW. Like my first trip out West, the mountains caused my eyes to pop, and my jaw to fall. I've never seen anything quite like the Canadian Rockies. They're strangely frightening and homey at the same time. I feel at home when I smell the fir trees and scared stupid when I drive along the foot of these awesome beasts we call mountains, feeling that I could be swallowed whole without anyone noticing. There's nothing quite like being there.

> **Is there a great trip that you've always wanted to take? Where do you want to go? Why? What would it take to make that trip happen?**

♥
First Year Teaching

My goal when I was finishing up my year at teachers' college was to get a job as soon as possible. I wanted to feel somewhat settled going into the summer. I wanted to enjoy the good weather without worrying about whether I would have a paycheck in September. After passing a generic school board interview, I was "recommended for hire" in York Region where Nick and I would be moving into a new home. My friend's sister, who was already working for that school board, gave me the vacancy list. After glancing through it for a week or so, Nick encouraged me to start making some calls. I decided to start calling about part-time positions. After everything I had gone through with anxiety and panic, I didn't feel like I could handle a full-time job in my first year of teaching.

I got an interview for a half-time kindergarten position at a school in a small town about an hour away from our apartment in the city. I was so excited about the principal's interest in interviewing me, that I was blind to the fact that it would take so long to get there. True, Nick and I would be moving a little closer to the school in a few months, but it was still not an enviable distance to drive once winter began and snow covered the roads.

Upon discovering the distance I was going to travel, even the principal tried to discourage me from coming for the interview.

"Are you sure you want to take a job so far from home?" he cautioned.

"Oh, no problem," I answered. "Besides, we've bought a house in Markham, so it won't be that bad."

I drove out the next morning during rush hour so I could see what it would really be like. There was quite a bit of traffic, but it did not deter me. I arrived all smiles, and answered all of his questions superbly. He took me for a tour of the school, introduced me to some teachers, and dropped me off in one of the kindergarten classrooms so that I could get a taste of what it would be like next year. When I returned to his office, he offered me the job. I was elated, and accepted the offer.

To this day, my year teaching in that school is like a badge of honor. The town is known to be rough around the edges, but I did not know this when I accepted the job. When I started working, I began to understand how it got its reputation.

My class consisted of 14 boys and 5 girls, a split junior/senior kindergarten. It was a nice small class, but the number of boys compared to girls made for an interesting mix of energy. I was constantly dealing with misbehavior. There was some extreme poverty in the town, and a disproportionate number of broken homes. But there were also a number of middle-class families that had moved far out of the city to the small town so that they could enjoy spacious homes and swimming pools for a fraction of the price it would have cost them in Toronto. Some kids came to school dirty, others in Roots dresses and pigtails. When the principal retired half way through the year, his speech included this memorable line: "If you can teach in this small town, you can teach anywhere."

Because teaching and having my own class was another new experience, my anxiety was high from the start. The night before the first day of school, I didn't really sleep. I woke up at 5:30 to get in the shower. I was so weak that I could barely hold up the hair dryer. I was so scared. I wanted to call a substitute teacher – *for the first day of school!* I wondered if it had ever been done. I was afraid that I'd pass out in the car on the way there. I was afraid that I'd pass out at school. I was almost certain that I wouldn't make it through the day. When Nick walked me down to the parking garage to say goodbye, he hugged me and I nearly broke into tears. His love was so powerful and so contrary to what I was giving myself that it was overwhelming. I got into the car. I drove half-way and stopped at a gas station to go to the washroom. I got to school with very little time to spare.

Before the bell rang, I saw the kids beginning to gather outside my door. I went outside to greet them. I felt like I was going to pass out. I saw one little blond boy crying, so I bent down to talk to him. I was so grateful to not have to stand vertically that I remained in a crouched position a little longer, trying to calm him. The bell rang. I led my class inside.

The year proceeded much like the first day, though perhaps not as extreme. I didn't like my job. I didn't like my school. I didn't like where it was. I made only one friend and I was so full of on-again-off-again anxiety that I didn't know what to do with myself. Thankfully, I only worked every other day, so the one-hour commute was not so terrible. Thankfully, I had a lot of supportive parents that volunteered in my classroom. Thankfully, I had a teacher-librarian that sympathized with me. Thankfully, I got a transfer at the end of the year to a school much closer to home.

I took thirteen days off that first year. I was allowed ten with pay, so I took three without. Most of the days I missed were because of my anxiety. One was a moving day, one was for a family function. The rest I took off because I was weak, nauseous, palpitating, short of breath, or some combination of those four. Sometimes, I went to work despite feeling those things. Sometimes I felt better as the day passed. Sometimes I felt worse. Once, I was on the verge of a panic attack, so I went home early.

I was still very much in the "why me?" phase. Still

searching desperately for solutions, and still not satisfied with what I was digging up. I visited my herbalist repeated times. I saw an Employee Assistance Provider for counselling. Sometimes I felt better, but never great. I was still searching for that strong Bonnie that had disappeared in the summer of '98.

> **What are some work or school-related concerns that you have that are not grounded in reality? Are you doing a great job, but still fear you'll be fired? Make a list of concerns related to work, and then write why it's okay to let those worries go.**

♥
Home Sweet Home

Shortly after Nick and I got married, we started looking for a house. Our families and cultures supported this kind of a move. Owning rather than renting was considered "putting money into your own pocket instead of someone else's." We looked at one or two new home developments outside the city, and settled on one that we liked in Markham, near the quaint town of Unionville. The housing market would not charge forward for at least two years, so we really got our pick of properties. We settled on a small detached house on a pie-shaped lot across from a small park.

Something that I hadn't yet figured out was that change and anxiety do not quite get along. I signed myself up for another move, yet didn't realize that it would be more stressful to me than to the average person.

Less than half-way through my first year teaching, we got possession of our home. I was very happy because it cut twenty minutes off my commute to work. I was happy to take a day off work for the move.

On the day we got the keys, I remember my mother-in-law bringing over her vacuum cleaner and asking me if I knew how to use the attachments to get into the corners. I meticulously went over each and every square centimeter, despite how I was feeling. I was feeling terrible – typically weak, nervous, and nauseous. I didn't enjoy the celebratory glass of champagne nearly as much as the others, because I was so overwhelmed with my symptoms.

Over the next few days, I was in moving flux. Surrounded by boxes and wanting everything to be perfect before sunset, I endured another round of anxiety and couldn't wait for it to feel like home so I could feel settled.

♥

Dr. Simpson

In the spring of my first year teaching, I was experiencing heart palpitations, nausea, lack of energy – the same routine all over again. Nick had not been working for three months, we had a new home and were surviving on a half-time salary. Even a "normal" person would feel anxious about that, I suppose. Once again feeling scared and convinced that there must be something physically wrong with me, I went to a local medical clinic where I was hoping to find a doctor that knew something the first twenty I had consulted didn't.

The doctor did a quick physical, and as far as he could tell, there wasn't anything physically wrong with me. Then, he did what most doctors do not take the time to do – he asked lots of questions that went well beyond the usual "any diseases run in your family?" He asked: What was it like growing up in my family? Where was I in the birth order? Was I a high achiever? How did I do in school? How did my parents react to my grades? I could tell that he was trying to get the *whole* picture, not just the biological one.

"How happy would you say you are?" Dr. Simpson asked.

"Well, what do you mean, on a scale of one to ten?" I stalled, answering in the form of a question.

"I don't know... I guess about a seven."

"Hmmm."

Dr. Simpson thought I was probably overrating my own happiness.

"I think you'd *like* it to be a seven, but I don't think it's really a seven," he explained.

"Oh."

When I got home, I went over the play-by-play of the appointment with Nick, including how impressed I'd been with the doctor taking the time to get to know the whole me. When I got to the part about Dr. Simpson thinking I'd overrated my own happiness, I started to weep. Suddenly, an unanswered voice deep within me started to call, and it wanted to be heard. When it spoke, it talked about travel.

Before I had moved into my apartment in the city, I had been planning to go on a tour of Israel. It was a pricey tour for young professionals, but I had the money in savings, and was willing to spend it to fulfill a dream. Going by myself was also part of the appeal. However, when the apartment came up, I decided to spend the money on rent instead. The trip never happened, but I guess the need to do it remained. Now I was smart enough to listen.

My travel voice talked aloud about going to Europe, Africa, Israel...it didn't seem to matter too much where – it just wanted me to *go*. While it was frightening to realize that I wasn't as happy as I thought I was, it was also cathartic to cry and begin to make plans to change, if only in my head to start.

That night, Nick turned to me in bed and said something that I am sure came straight from God.

"Bon, somewhere along the line, you've lost your strength. You've gotta go somewhere – to live or whatever to get that kick-ass Bonnie back."

I couldn't believe my ears. It was exactly what I

needed to hear, though I had no idea that I needed to hear it. I felt set free. Being married had changed how I dreamed, and how I thought about options and plans. One of my greatest qualities, and one that comes quite naturally to me, is being a devoted, affectionate and committed wife. The problem is that my devotedness to the role of wife means that at times I can quite unintentionally take me away from *me*.

The next few weeks were, at the same time, wonderful and scary. I started to talk to my close friends about my epiphany after the trip to the doctor's, about not being as happy as I thought I was. The friends I talked to had known me since I was thirteen. They knew I had been suffering for three years with *something*. They were eager to hear about my epiphany, and to help me get to the next stage of healing. Keira, Sunny, Brian, Jen and Nick were willing ears and I was so grateful for the love, caring, and wisdom they shared and continue to share.

My friend Brian, who had just returned from ten months of studying and traveling through Southeast Asia, was extremely supportive of my travel idea. We talked on the phone and then went to a ball game and talked some more. The bravery he showed by living half-way around world in a foreign country was an inspiration to me. It made me feel more confident that my resurrected dream was not crazy and that indeed it could come true.

My friend Sunny and I went out for a bite to eat, and I remember exactly what she expressed. *Happiness is found within. Everything you need is right here in Toronto, you don't need to go traveling to find it.* Because of Sunny's deep spiritual beliefs, I valued her insight, but I still wanted to go. I knew that I needed to travel, and if the yearning was returning over and over again, it likely meant something.

My best friend Jen asked me the big questions. I shared my fears about not being independent-enough of a person, and she helped me to ask myself some important though frightening questions. I began to wonder whether I rushed into getting married, denying myself the "stand on your own two feet" confidence that so many women have. Jen asked whether Nick and I might have rushed into buying a house so soon after getting married. Her and her husband were still renting an apartment and planning to live across the country in Vancouver for a couple of years before they settled down.

A pain-in-the-ass problem about best friends is that they know you well enough to usually be right. While I would never trade being married to Nick, I could see how assuming the responsibility of owning a house so soon after getting married automatically ties up finances and dreams that might otherwise have come to fruition. Being married and a homeowner might have contributed to putting my travel dreams on the back burner.

I decided that I would start researching travel options. At the travel agency, I picked up all sorts of brochures, and then went to the library to sign out videos and travel books. Africa looked great. Going on a safari had always been a dream of mine. Alternatively, I had never been to Austria or Eastern Europe, which looked equally interesting. Though I didn't realize my trip until over a year later, the important thing was that the seed was planted. An important voice had received some critical air time.

Is there something that you've always wanted to do that you haven't got around to doing? How would you feel if you finally did it? What steps can you take towards that goal? Is there some small way that you can step towards that goal today?

PART III
RECOVERY

Recovery

♥
The Clinic

My recovery really fast-forwarded when I started seeing a therapist in a place that specialized in helping people with anxiety and depression related disorders. It was a big relief, after all my searching, to finally walk through the door and be told that it would be possible to return to a 'normal' life.

The Clinic in downtown Toronto was recommended to me by an Employee Assistance Provider (EAP) that Nick had been seeing. He had become certifiably miserable over his job, and I had convinced him that seeing a therapist might help soothe his sleepless nights and stomach aches. After listening patiently to his story, Amanda, his therapist, understood that some of Nick's stress was as a result of his wife's problem with anxiety and panic. Because I didn't feel well enough to work full time, Nick was unable to entertain other career options such as going back to school to become a teacher. I was working half-time as a kindergarten teacher and didn't feel like I could promise anything more than that. Amanda asked Nick to bring me along for his next session so that we could sort some things out together.

The answers to our prayers often come in the strangest ways. I had been praying for years for help with getting better, and here it came in the form of my *husband's* therapist.

Amanda was the first therapist to draw tears. I felt like she was only on Nick's side, which is what he had feared. When she asked whether there was a reason I couldn't work full time to support Nick in his plans to be a teacher, I felt attacked. Granted, I am a sensitive person. Then Amanda asked whether I would be willing to attack my anxiety problem with a proven cure. And that is how I heard about The Clinic.

While I was ecstatic at the prospect of being cured, I couldn't help but be frustrated that it took a Toronto 'Bay Street' therapist to identify both my problem *and* the solution. Why didn't more professionals in the field of healing know about panic and anxiety? Why was this proven solution so difficult to find? Nonetheless, I was glad to finally be on my way.

During my initial consultation at The Clinic with the supervising psychologist, Dr. Randy Katz, I was given the opportunity to describe the events of the past four years, beginning with the panic attack in Paris. Dr. Katz looked me in the eye and told me with absolute certainty that I had panic disorder. I felt relief and yet still a hint of denial.

Dr. Katz explained that panic attacks are so traumatic that people usually tailor their thoughts and behaviors to avoid having another one. They avoid the places that are associated with their panic attacks. Some people become agoraphobic – they avoid leaving the house at all because they believe something 'out there' will make it more likely that a panic attack will occur. A person's home is their safe place. It is predictable, and comfortable, so we want to stay there. That sounded a lot like the summer that I was literally house-bound because of my fears.

I had never really thought of my thoughts and behaviors in the way that Dr. Katz had described. The more I thought about it though, the more I realized that I was very careful about avoiding situations or feelings that might instigate a panic attack. I had created a new world around that fear. I was careful not to plan too much in one day in case I felt drained and more vulnerable to an attack. I avoided and feared very hot and humid environments, because I was afraid that I would feel like I couldn't breathe.

I finally came to accept that I did have panic disorder. I, a normal, average, intelligent person had a mental illness. And if I had one, I wondered who else out there just like me had one too.

♥
Relaxation

Dr. Katz set me up with one of the young therapists working in his clinic. I met with Laurel Gordon for the first time in January of 2002. Laurel spent the first session gathering background information. I already remembered Dr. Solomon's warning that my subconscious would try to find something about the therapist or the setting that it didn't like in a subversive attempt to usurp the counseling process. *I would come back for the second appointment whether or not my subconscious tried to convince me otherwise!*

At first, I saw Laurel every two weeks. Early in the therapy process, Laurel introduced me to one of the main strategies people with panic and anxiety need to calm down and relax: ten minutes of quiet, unadulterated, intentional daily relaxation.

The first few months of my therapy started with ten minutes of guided relaxation. Laurel read a relaxation script while I sat with my eyes closed, following her instructions. For five minutes, I practiced deep breathing and developed an awareness of where I was holding tension in my body. I was guided to draw breaths deep into my belly. For the next five minutes, I practiced progressive muscle relaxation. Beginning with my feet, I was told to tense then relax various body parts, holding the tension for about five seconds before releasing. I did this several times, with different muscle groups, moving upwards towards my head. After time, I noticed that I held most of my tension in my upper back and shoulders, so we tailored the relaxation script to suit my needs. I tensed those muscles twice before moving on to the next muscle group.

The immediate effects of this relaxation practice were extraordinary. When the ten minutes ended and I opened my eyes, I felt as if I had taken a nice long nap. It was both refreshing *and* effective at reducing my level of anxiety.

Laurel encouraged me to practice this relaxation routine every day. She made me an audio tape so that I could do it at home.

The relaxation routine had an enormous impact on my state of anxiety. Once I treated it as a necessary part of my recovery, it had the effect of making me more relaxed in general. I have included Laurel's script at the end of my story (Appendix A). I highly recommend daily relaxation practice as a vital part of recovery from panic disorder.

♥
Thought Records

The second component that was essential in my recovery from panic disorder was learning how to record and challenge my negative thought patterns in Thought Records. David Burns describes the thought record process in *Feeling Good*. He states: "Your negative thoughts, or cognitions, are the most frequently overlooked symptoms

*My Sample Thought Record

Situation	Emotion(s)	Automatic Thought(s)	Alternative Response	Outcome
Describe the actual event, stream of thoughts, daydream, or recollection leading to unpleasant emotion. (Who, what when, where).	1. Specify sad, anxious, angry, etc. 2. Rate 0-100.	1. Write automatic thought(s) preceding emotion(s). What was going through my mind just before I started to feel bad? Any images? 2. Rate 0-100%.	1. Write rational response or alternative response to automatic thought(s). 2. Rate 0-100%.	1. Specify subsequent emotion(s). 2. Rate 0-100.
It is Sunday evening before going back to work. I am lying down watching television and I am feeling very weak.	Anxious 75 Fearful 70	1. I am a bad teacher. 2. I cannot control my class. 3. I'll never be good at this job.	I am not a bad teacher; I am a beginning teacher. I cannot be expected to be perfect at this complex job right away. There are many things that I am doing well; I will try to accept that I am still learning.	Anxious 40 Fearful 35

*This thought record was given to me by my therapist. It is adapted from:
Beck. A. T. Rush A. J., Shaw B. F. & Emery. G. (1979). *Cognitive Therapy for Depression*. The Guilford Press: New York.
Greenberger, D. & Padesky, C. (1995). *Mind Over Mood: A Cognitive Therapy Treatment Manual for Clients*. The Guilford Press: New York

of your [anxiety]."[12] In his book, Burns writes about how to recover from depression, but the same process can be successfully applied to recovery from panic disorder and anxiety.

There are five columns in the thought record I learned to use. I have included a copy of one of my own thought records to help you follow along. In addition, a blank thought record has been provided in Appendix B for you to photocopy.

In the first column titled *Situation*, I describe in detail the situation in which I find myself feeling poorly. For example: "It is Sunday evening before going back to work. I am lying down watching television and I am feeling very weak." This column is strictly a description of who, what, where, and when.

In the second column titled *Emotion(s)*, I list the emotions that I am feeling. This takes a bit of thought. On the Sunday night before going back to work, I felt "anxious" and "fearful".

Next, I rate my listed emotions on a scale from one to 100. This rating process involves some valuable learning. When I first started doing the thought records, I would rate my emotions very high. Laurel helped me to realize that a rating of 100 for an emotion like anxiety meant that I was in the middle of a full-blown panic attack. Usually, this wasn't the case. I soon began to rate my emotions in a way that was more reflective of reality. This was an important learning point. Seeing the situation as it actually was, and not inflating it in my mind was part of the process of changing my thought patterns.

---

[12] *Feeling Good: The New Mood Therapy.* David Burns. (1980). New York: Avon Books.

Cognitive Patterns*

*These cognitive patterns were given to me by my therapist. They are adapted from: Burns, David D. (1980). Feeling Good: The New Mood Therapy. New York: Avon Books.

1. **All-or-Nothing Thinking:** You see thinks in black-and white categories. If your performance falls short of perfect, you see yourself as a total failure.

2. **Overgeneralization**: You see a single negative event as a never-ending pattern of defeat.

3. **Mental Filter:** You pick out a single negative detail and dwell on it exclusively so that your vision of all reality becomes darkened, like the drop of ink that colors the entire beaker of water.

4. **Disqualifying the Positive:** You reject positive experiences by insisting they "don't count" for some reason or other. In this way you can maintain a negative belief that is contradicted by your everyday experiences.

5. **Jumping to Conclusions:** You make a negative interpretation even though there are no definite facts that convincingly support your conclusion.
a. *Mind Reading:* You arbitrarily conclude that someone is reacting negatively to you, and you don't bother to check this out.
b. *Fortune Telling:* You anticipate that things will turn out badly, and you feel convinced that your prediction is an already-established fact.

6. **Magnification (Catastrophizing) or Minimization:** You exaggerate the importance of things (such as your goof-up or someone else's achievement), or you inappropriately shrink things until they appear tiny (your own desirable qualities or the other fellow's imperfections). This is also called the "binocular trick".

7. **Emotional Reasoning:** You assume that your negative emotions necessarily reflect the way things really are: "I feel it, therefore it must be true."

8. **"Should Statements":** You try to motivate yourself with "shoulds" and "shouldn'ts", as if you had to be whipped and punished before you could be expected to do anything. "Musts" and "oughts" are also offenders. The emotional consequence is guilt. When you direct "should" statements toward others, you feel anger, frustration, and resentment.

9. **Labeling and Mislabeling:** This is an extreme form of overgeneralization. Instead of describing your error, you attach a negative label to yourself: "I'm a loser." When someone else's behavior rubs you the wrong way, you attach a negative label to him: "He's an idiot." Mislabeling involves describing an event with language that is highly colored and emotionally loaded.

10. **Personalization:** You see yourself as the cause of some negative external event for which, in fact, you were not primarily responsible.

The third column of the thought record, titled *Automatic Thought(s)*, is where the work of change and healing really begins. Automatic Thoughts contain the words of our inner critic. These thoughts seem to sneak up on us. We don't even know our automatic thoughts exist most of the time. By spending time discovering how we talk to ourselves, we can see how our internal dialogue is often hurtful. Harmful automatic thoughts affect us negatively on physical, mental and spiritual levels. My automatic thoughts were the root cause of my physical symptoms such as fatigue, dizziness, lack of appetite, and heart palpitations. When I was completing my thought record that Sunday night, I realized that my automatic thoughts were: "I am a bad teacher," "I cannot control my class" and "I'll never feel confident at work". Pretty strong statements. I didn't take a survey of my colleagues or ask my supervisor, but I was convinced those were true – until I began to dissect them, and turn them around.

Laurel guided me in an analysis of my automatic thoughts. She gave me a list of Cognitive Patterns to match with each of the automatic thoughts I listed. The Cognitive Patterns are distorted ways of thinking typical of those suffering from anxiety or depression. They describe ways in which our minds bend reality.

Referring back to my thought record, my first automatic thought, "I am a bad teacher," reflects *All-or-Nothing Thinking* (I see my teaching only as good or bad, nothing in-between). It also reflects *Disqualifying the Positive*, because I disqualify all the positive experiences I have had with my students. My thought also reflects *Emotional Reasoning*. I felt like I was a bad teacher, so therefore I reasoned I was. I was also guilty of *Labeling*, calling myself a bad teacher, because I attached a negative label to myself.

The next step Laurel taught me is not on the thought record page. On the reverse side of the page, I write one of the automatic thoughts as a title. Then below the title, I make a T-shaped column with "Evidence For" and "Evidence Against" as the sub-headings. Here is an example:

I am a bad teacher

Evidence For	*Evidence Against*
• I do not have my day plan set three days in advance like I am supposed to • I cannot control my class • I don't have any long-range plans or units	• I have developed a good rapport with many of my students • I have had some compliments from my colleagues • I have special education students, so the successes are slower and less frequent • My students look forward to drama and ask for more • My students enjoy cooking and ask for more • I feel like I'm helping at least some of them

Usually, the evidence against my automatic thoughts was more substantial than the evidence for them. Completing this chart was an important process in challenging my often-damaging automatic thoughts. I usually completed this t-chart for the strongest statement in my list of automatic thoughts.

The fourth column in the thought record is where I generate alternative responses to my automatic thoughts. I did not complete this column with my therapist until I had become quite good at columns one through three. She made sure to carefully guide me through each and every step of the process, not rushing forward too quickly.

Alternative responses became easier to generate after doing the t-chart on the back of the thought record. In fact, alternative responses began to sneak into the *Evidence Against* column. Laurel also introduced me to a list of Dispute Handles (see next page) as a guide to generating alternative responses. In the case of the statement *"I am a bad teacher,"* my alternative response was: "I am not a bad teacher. I am a beginning teacher. I cannot be expected to be perfect at this complex job right away. There are many things that I am doing well. I will try to accept that I am still learning." I then continued to come up with equally rational responses for all my automatic thoughts. Sometimes, an overarching alternative response can cover more than one automatic thought.

The fifth and final column of the thought record is where I reassess the emotions I was feeling before I did the thought record. Each of the original emotions from column two is copied over, and re-rated on a scale of one to 100. The hope is that the cognitive process involved in completing the thought record will lessen the degree of negative feeling or emotion that was present before. For example, after completing the thought record, my feeling of anxiety decreased from an initial rating of 70 down to 45.

The thought records WORK. They seem stupid and mundane at times, but the exercise of doing them whenever bad feelings arise sets in motion a different way of thinking. People struggling with anxiety have great difficulty generating alternative responses on their own. They must go through the thought record process to help alternative responses come more naturally. New neural pathways must be forged and reinforced repeatedly. The results are not immediate, but they come. I am proof of that.

> **Dispute Handles***
>
> Do I know for certain that _____ will happen?
> Am I 100% sure of these awful consequences?
> What evidence do I have that _____?
> Does _____ have to equal or lead to_____?
> Do I have a crystal ball?
> What is the worst that could happen? How bad is that?
> Could there be any other explanations?
> What is the likelihood that _____?
> Is _____ really so important or consequential?
> Does _____'s opinion reflect that of everyone else?
> Is _____ really so important that my entire future resides with its outcome?
>
> ---
>
> *These Dispute Handles were given to me by my therapist. They are adapted from:
> 1) Beck, A. T., Rush, A. J., Shaw B. F. & Emery, G. (1979). <u>Cognitive Therapy for Depression</u>. New York: The Guilford Press.
> 2) Burns, D. (1989). <u>The Feeling Good Handbook</u>. New York: Plume.
> 3) Greenberger, D. & Padesky, C. (1995). <u>Mind Over Mood: A Cognitive Therapy Treatment Manual for Clients</u>. New York: The Guilford Press.

♥
Kia ora

I had been seeing Laurel for about four or five months when I decided that I was finally going to make one of my dreams come true. Well before I was married, I wanted to go on a big solo trip to Israel. After the visit to Dr. Simpson when he suggested I wasn't as happy as I

Recovery

thought I was, I realized that traveling anywhere would be just fine, as long as I did it by myself. I decided that I would apply for a year-long special leave of absence from teaching to allow me to travel. I had thought about Europe, but I knew it was very expensive, and had already been to several countries there. I decided on New Zealand. I reasoned that it was small enough to conquer in a relatively short period of time, and Kiwis have the reputation of being very friendly.

My trip, though a dream-come-true, was not without its rough spots. I decided to stop in on my old friend the Rocky Mountains on my way out west. At the hostel in Lake Louise, I took a yoga class one morning. About ten minutes into the class, my body went into shut-down. It felt like one more downward dog was going to send me into a full-fledged panic attack. I sat for a moment, and then slipped out of the class. Luckily, I recognized the reasons behind my strange feeling. The normal anxiety I was feeling about traveling to the other side of the globe by myself had stored itself in my body, and the yoga class forced it out. I went to a pay phone and called Nick.

Before long, I was bawling. It wasn't that I didn't want to go through with the trip; I just needed someone I trusted deeply to talk to about my fears. Nick reassured me that he had had similar feelings before setting off to Europe on his own several years before. He assured me that my anxiety would abate as I became more comfortable with traveling. I was so glad to hear that.

Still, my first few weeks in New Zealand were no party. I was out of my comfort zone. Staying mostly in hostels, I had to put up with lesser degrees of cleanliness, quiet and comfort than I was used to. I found it hard to adjust to not having a fridge or cupboard with all my favourite foods within arms' reach. One night during my first week, I was awoken by the shrieks a British girl, and then I saw a shadowy figure dart out of our dorm room. After the visit from the thief, I slept with one eye open for a while.

By the time I reached my fourth city, I was feeling weak, tired, confused, and actually quite miserable. I called Nick and broke down several times. I prayed. This was not what I had bargained for when I spent all my savings.

Aug 17/02

I HAVE HAD IT WITH THESE FUCKING <u>HOSTELS!</u> I hate them! I hate them! If it's not one thing it's another. Noisy <u>OR</u> no fucking bathroom or NO FUCKING NO FUCKING NO FUCKING <u>HEAT</u> FOR GOD'S SAKE. Goodbye I've had it! I was actually feeling BETTER thank you very much and then there's no FUCKING <u>heat!!!!</u> I am ready to I don't know what. 3 questions before I agree to stay ANYWHERE:

1) DO YOU HAVE HEATERS THAT FUCKING WORK!!

2) Are your bathrooms fucking INSIDE?

3) Is it a zoo or can we expect some level of quiet there???

Fuck it. Fuck this. I don't know what to do anymore. I can't can't can't go on like this. Can't. It's too much. Fuck this.

August 18, 2002

Switch. No (or less) hostels. No outdoor bathrooms. Bonnie has had enough (evidence: the CONSTANT weeping of the last 3 to 4 days.) Love it or hate it, that's the way I am. I can't hostel it. I can't do it. I sort of knew this going in, but thought I could get by. I can't. And really

really really not enjoying my trip is a failure I'm not willing to absorb. No way. I looked forward to this too much. I did not spend all this money to have a crappy time. No no no way. I am going to enjoy at least most of my time – most of the rest of my time.

Which is not to say I won't get lonely and homesick. BUT I will not spend the majority of my energy simply surviving – namely: eating, sleeping. It ceased to be enjoyable when I spent my energy surviving or worrying about the quality of my living quarters. Love it. It's the only way. Love the fact that I can't "bottom barrel" it. I am a high-class (or medium-class?) girl, and that's just the way it is. Just the way it is. I love it. I may not be able to afford it, but I love it.

From that moment, I started to feel better. I booked more hotels and less hostels, a couple of domestic flights, and shortened my trip by two weeks so that I could afford it.

♥
Cape Reinga

One of the most amazing places I visited in New Zealand was Cape Reinga. It lies at the northernmost tip of New Zealand's North Island.

I was on a bus tour that hit the popular tourist sites north of Paihia, a beach town about two hours north of Auckland. As the bus approached the Cape, the landscape became vast and desolate. A few sheep or dairy farms spotted the land, but what was striking was the incredible green rolling hills and the vast ocean spilling out in every direction from where the land dropped off.

As the bus pulled up to the small parking lot, the

driver explained that Cape Reinga is a sacred site. The Maori people believe that the deceased leave Aotearoa, the Maori name for New Zealand, at Cape Reinga and succumb to the blue ocean. At an island far off shore, barely visible from the Cape, the spirits resurface, take one last look at their homeland, and then disappear back into the world of water and spirit forevermore.

Standing at the edge of the Cape, it is ocean as far as the eye can see. Cape Reinga sits where the Pacific Ocean from the east meets the Tasman Sea from the west. The crests of waves from the two bodies of water actually collide mid-sea. It was just amazing. Without question, a sacred place.

Despite the extreme wind, I wanted to stay there all day. The view was just spectacular. I felt like I was God looking down on all that is good in the world, and smiling. I felt like I was witness to all the glory that is God while I sat high atop the ocean and the waves and the vastness of the water.

At one point, I stood looking over the west side of the cliffs and tears started coming to my eyes. The beauty of the movement of the waves as they hit the rocky shore was suddenly the most beautiful thing I had ever seen.

♥
Maintenance

My goal when I entered therapy with Laurel was to feel like I could work full-time. Until then, I didn't feel strong enough mentally or physically to do that. It took exactly one year of therapy to reach my goal. To me, it seemed reasonable that it took one year to change twenty-eight years of maladaptive thinking.

I was very happy with my results. I continued to see Laurel once every two or three weeks for another year and a half. I also called her whenever a crisis would come up. Laurel is very proud of our success together, especially proud of my determination and hard work.

Recovery from panic and anxiety has come because I have incorporated my therapy into my day-to-day routine. I often focus on my breathing. Shallow breaths are a signal that I am under stress. I still use a relaxation tape to help me unwind once in a while. I incorporate the thought record process much more automatically into my way of thinking, but that does not mean that I never do thought records. Sometimes, it is necessary for me to go through the process again to turn a maladaptive thought on its head.

Laurel has also helped me to recognize my triggers. There are situations that will predispose me to anxiety or to panic attacks. Stressful times at work or home, very hot days and highly emotional events are all potential triggers for me. When I am exposed to these things, I try very hard to use my deep breathing techniques and to recognize any thoughts that might cause me to spiral downwards. I call on my support network when I can, and I use personal evidence to convince me that *I will be okay!*

♥
Are you ever "cured"?

I am not perfect. I admit that there are times that I think I am slipping back into that person who was crippled by anxiety.

Just last year, when my paternal grandfather was dying, I freaked out. I didn't think I could handle my job as a full-time teacher and being a supportive granddaughter. I thought I would faint at the funeral. But I reminded myself that I have a host of coping mechanisms now that I didn't have before. So I did thought records, I went to see my therapist, I went for a massage, I prayed and I talked to friends. I made it through. To my surprise, I even delivered the eulogy at the funeral.

When life gets really stressful like that, I begin to think that I am not much different from that woman who had her first panic attack in Paris. But I am. My ability to cope with stress and with uncomfortable situations has strengthened. I am proud to carry a diverse tool box of coping mechanisms with me wherever I go.

♥

Conclusion

Marianne Williamson and Caroline Myss, among others, say that we act out of only two emotions: Love or Fear. I am grateful that I have gone through the process of healing from panic disorder because I have learned to lead with love more than ever before.

Some people who I share my story with ask me why I think it happened. Why did I get panic attacks? Why did I suffer from anxiety? Why did it start when I was 24 years old?

I answer that I was called by my Higher Self to heal parts of my soul. I was with an unconditionally loving partner when the pot began to stir, and I suppose I was ready to begin learning the lessons I needed to learn to move forward and grow. As time passes, I receive more and more insights into those questions of why.

If we say only one prayer, it is supposed to be "Thank You". I am grateful beyond measure because this process of healing has helped me to become a better me. I am grateful to be more loving and to be living with less fear. I am grateful for the miracles that have passed since I first chose to believe that they can indeed happen. I am grateful for a closer relationship to Spirit, to God, to my Higher Self, to Angels and to the Universe. I am grateful for how I have grown in my relationships with others. I am grateful that I feel brave enough to share my story with you. I am grateful for believing that you can heal because I have.

Appendix A

Relaxation and Progressive Relaxation Script*

*Script is adapted from:
Bourne, E.J. (2000). The Anxiety and Phobia Workbook. Oakland: New Harbinger Publications Inc. 3rd Edition.

And is based on the principles of
Wolpe, J. (1958). Psychotherapy by Reciprocal Inhibition. Stanford: Stanford University Press.
and
Beck, A.T., Rush, A. J., Shaw, B. F., Emery, G. (1979). Cognitive Therapy of Depression. New York: Guilford Inc.

Have this script recorded onto a tape or CD so that you can play it back without having to refer to this page. Your therapist can do this for you. Alternatively, record it yourself or ask a friend or family member who has a relaxing voice to record it for you. Bourne suggests alternative tapes for relaxation in Appendix 3 (p.431) of The Anxiety and Phobia Workbook.

Part One: Relaxation

- Find a place where you can lie down or sit down. A place that is comfortable for you. Feel free to alter the exercise in any way that enables you to feel more relaxed.

- Note the level of tension you're feeling. Then place one

hand on your abdomen right beneath your rib cage. In abdominal breathing, the diaphragm – the muscle that separates the lung cavity from the abdominal cavity – moves downward. In so doing, it causes the muscles surrounding the abdominal cavity to push outward.

• When you have taken in a full breath, pause for a moment and then exhale slowly through your nose or your mouth, depending on your preference. Be sure to exhale fully. As you exhale, allow your whole body to just let go (you might visualize your arms and legs going loose and limp like a rag doll).

• Do 10 slow, full abdominal breaths. Try to keep your breathing smooth and regular, without gulping in a big breath or letting your breath out all at once. It will help to slow down your breathing if you slowly count to 4 on the inhale and 4 on the exhale.

• Extend the exercise, if you wish, by doing 2 or 3 sets of abdominal breaths, for 5 minutes.

• If you start to feel light-headed while practicing, stop for 10-15 seconds, and then start again.

Part Two: Progressive Muscle Relaxation

• Gently close your eyes, uncross your arms and slide them to your sides with your palms up. Uncross your legs, and take a deep breath. All you have to do now is listen to my voice. Give yourself permission to forget all the concerns of the day. At any time during the exercise, you can come back to the room and open your eyes. At any point during the exercise, feel free to make any alterations to the exercise that enable you to become more relaxed.

• Now take a deep breath in as if a wave is coming

in to shore. And now exhale, as if the wave is being drawn out to sea.

• Now I would like you to focus on your feet. Point your toes downward so that you tense the muscles in your feet... Now release.

• Now focus on your calves. Point your feet downward so that you feel the tension in your calves...and release.

• Now shift your focus to your thighs. Press your thighs together so that you feel the tension in your thighs... And release. Notice the difference between tension and relaxation in these muscles.

• Now shift your focus to your abdomen. Tighten the muscles in your abdomen by sucking your belly button in as if it were to touch your spine... And release. Take a deep breath. Enjoy the pleasant sensations as relaxation begins to take place.

• Allow these muscles to continue relaxing while you shift your attention to your hands. Tighten your hands by making a fist. Feel the tension in your hands... And release.

• Now focus on your shoulders. Raise your shoulders towards your ears. Feel the muscles pull... And release.

• Focus on the muscles between your shoulder blades. Tense these muscles by sliding your shoulder blades toward each other... And release.

• Now shift your focus to your forehead. Tense the muscles in your forehead – you can do so by raising your eyebrows upward...And release. Let your muscles relax and allow the wave of relaxation to warm you.

Concentrate on your breathing. Take a deep breath in...and breathe out. Again, in...feel the air going into your lungs...and out. With each breath out you are becoming more and more relaxed. Gently let yourself continue breathing in whatever way feels comfortable and easy for you. And when you're ready, open your eyes and come back to the room.

*Blank Thought Record

Situation	Emotion(s)	Automatic Thought(s)	Alternative Response	Outcome
Describe the actual event, stream of thoughts, daydream, or recollection leading to unpleasant emotion. (Who, what when, where).	1. Specify sad, anxious, angry, etc. 2. Rate 0-100.	1. Write automatic thought(s) preceding emotion(s). What was going through my mind just before I started to feel bad? Any images? 2. Rate 0-100%.	1. Write rational response or alternative response to automatic thought(s). 2. Rate 0-100%.	1. Specify subsequent emotion(s). 2. Rate 0-100.

*This thought record was given to me by my therapist. It is adapted from:
Beck, A. T., Rush, A. J., Shaw B. F. & Emery, G. (1979). *Cognitive Therapy for Depression*. The Guilford Press: New York.
Greenberger, D. & Padesky, C. (1995). *Mind Over Mood: A Cognitive Therapy Treatment Manual for Clients*. The Guilford Press: New York

Annotated References

Here is a list of references that have helped me on my journey.

A Day of Rest: Creating A Spiritual Space in Your Week by Martha Whitmore Hickman. (1999). New York: Avon Books, Inc.
I don't care which religion we do or do not adhere to or rebel from. We all need a day of rest during our work week, whatever shape that might take. Easier said than done... But God took one, so why shouldn't we?

Anatomy of the Spirit: The Seven Stages of Power and Healing by Caroline Myss. (1996). New York: Crown Publishers.
Amazing, amazing, amazing, like Gary Zukav's The Seat of the Soul. *I wish I could write books like this! Caroline is an intuitive healer. In this book, she talks about how our health around the seven charkas is a reflection of our specific life issues.*

Archetypal Reiki: Spiritual, Emotional & Physical Healing (Book and Cards) by Dorothy May. (2000). Boston: Journey Editions.
This book and card set is interesting to play with, especially if you feel you need some direction with an issue.

A Return to Love: Reflections on the Principles of A Course in Miracles by Marianne Williamson. (1993). New York: HarperCollins.
This is the book that convinced me it's alright to ask for a miracle if you need one.

A Woman's Book of Life: The Biology, Psychology, and Spirituality of the Feminine Life Cycle by Joan Borysenko. (1996). New York: Riverhead Books.
Upon my friend Norm Jones' suggestion, I drove to Warren, Ohio to hear Joan speak, and bought this book there. She is wonderful.

Beyond Anxiety & Phobia: A Step-by-Step Guide to Lifetime Recovery by Edmund J. Bourne. (2001). Oakland, CA: New Harbinger Publications.
The author of The Anxiety and Phobia Workbook *strikes again with this holistic conclusion to his previous work. Excellent. Highly recommend it.*

Conversations With God, Book 1: An Uncommon Dialogue by Neale Donald Walsch. (1996). Viking Children's Books.
Automatic writing reveals God's voice. This book reveals many truths. Walsch asks all the right questions.

Death: The Final Stage of Growth by Elisabeth Kübler-Ross. (1975). New York: Touchstone.
Kübler-Ross' perspectives on death are intelligent, insightful, inspiring and sensitive. I highly recommend any of her books.

Diagnostic and Statistical Manual of Mental Disorders - Fourth Edition (DSM-IV). (1994). The American Psychiatric Association, Washington D.C.
This is the oft-cited bible of diagnosis in the psychiatric/psychological world. The symptoms of all anxiety-related disorders, including panic disorder are also mentioned in chapter one of Bourne's The Anxiety and Phobia Workbook.

Feeling Good: The New Mood Therapy by David D. Burns. (1980). New York: Avon Books.
This is a great book about cognitive behavioural therapy. It will give you an idea of what you have in store.

From Panic to Power: Proven Techniques to Calm Your Anxieties, Conquer Your Fears, and Put You in Control of Your Life by Lucinda Basset. (1995). New York: HarperCollins.
This book was recommended to me. If you struggle with anxiety or panic, you will find yourself in the pages of this book. It's uncanny. Not a replacement for therapy, but good to read nonetheless.

Give the Gift of Healing: A Concise Guide to Spiritual Healing by Rosemary Altea (book and tape). (1997). New York: Eagle Brook.
An amazing book that helped me at the beginning of my journey. Rosemary is a medium that uses her guide, Grey Eagle, to help her heal. Truths throughout.

Healing Spirit – a film by Hubert Schuurman. (1993). Montreal: National Film Board of Canada.
Frustrated with conventional medicine, many who suffer turn to prayer, meditation and spirit to find meaning in their lives and in their illnesses. Deepak Chopra and Dr. Bernie Siegel lend their wisdom. "To heal at the deepest level, you need to go into the pain," suggests Siegel.

How to Get What You Want and Want What You Have: A Practical and Spiritual Guide to Personal Success by John Gray. (1999). New York: HarperCollins.
Very inspiring and motivating, but not therapy. Use as a tool, not as a solution. Good section on meditation.

Illusions: The Adventures of a Reluctant Messiah by Richard Bach. (1989). Ballentine Books.
Recommended by my friend Norm Jones. I started to read it much after I bought it and I thought it was 'new age amazing'. A quick read, but great lessons.

Living Juicy: Daily Morsels for Your Creative Soul by SARK. (1994). Berkley: Celestial Arts.
This book was a gift. The inside dedication reads: HAPPY BIRTHDAY BONNIE!! Here are some wonderful ideas and reminders for your self-prescribed "BONNIE YEAR" which I find so exciting and inspirational. This book is actually not just for the "BONNIE YEAR" it's for the entire "BONNIE LIFE" Enjoy! Love, Your Friend, Tamara. I couldn't have said it better myself.

Lucky Man: A Memoir by Michael J. Fox. (2002). New York: Hyperion.
I was a big Michael J. Fox fan when I was young. I could relate to his story about coping with Parkinson's Disease. He was going along thinking everything was going okay until suddenly it

wasn't. It ended up being the best thing that ever happened to him.

One Day My Soul Just Opened Up: 40 Days and 40 Nights Toward Spiritual Strength and Personal Growth by Iyanla Vanzant. (1998). New York: Fireside.
Part inspiration, part journal, this book allows you to read and then reflect each day (or night) for 40 days. If you only get to the 10th day, it will have been worthwhile. It's a great way to reflect, grow and learn.

On Grief and Dying: Understanding the Soul's Journey by Diane Stein. (1996). Freedom, CA: The Crossing Press, Inc.
The first book I read to help me cope with the death of my grandfather. It was very comforting.

Reaching to Heaven: A Spiritual Journey Through Life and Death by James Van Praagh. (1999). New York: Signet. (Also: Talking to Heaven by the same author).
James Van Praagh is a spiritual medium who contacts people who have passed on, like John Edward on the show <u>Crossing Over</u>. Van Praagh's books are full of interesting stories that will make you a believer of life on the other side.

The Anxiety and Phobia Workbook: Third Edition by Edmund J. Bourne. (2000). Oakland, CA, New Harbinger Publications.
As far as I'm concerned, this is the bible of anxiety disorders. I'm not sure why I didn't start reading it sooner. I was probably in denial. Hopefully you won't be and will pick up a copy of this heavyweight at your local library or bookstore. Bourne is an expert, and his writing and research are bang-on.

The Bodacious Book of Succulence: Daring to Live Your Succulent Wild Life! by SARK. (1998). New York: Fireside.
I love SARK. Her books are pretty. She guides us simply, realistically, and encourages us to be accepting of ourselves. And she inspires. Highly recommended.

The Celestine Prophecy: An Adventure by James Redfield. (1993). New York: Warner Books.
One of the first new age books I read. Great lessons.

The Life You Were Born to Live: A Guide to Finding Your Life Purpose by Dan Millman. (1993). Tiburon, CA: H J Kramer Inc.
A must-have and a must-read. If you are on 'the path', you will find yourself in this book. Based on life numbers, Dan's descriptions are bang-on accurate. Laws at the end of the book help get you through rough spots. GET IT!

The Seat of the Soul by Gary Zukav. (1989). New York: Fireside.
I have re-read parts of this book on many occasions. What great truths. It's the kind of book that you pick up off your shelf and open to the right page. Gary's got an amazingly patient disposition. He's been on Oprah, and he talks about how he used to be an angry man. Hard to believe.

The Tao of Pooh by Benjamin Hoff. (1982). New York: Dutton.
All about Taoism, from the perspective of Winnie-The-Pooh. A wonderful philosophy to adopt, or at least read about.

Transformation Soup: Healing for the Splendidly Imperfect by SARK. (2000). New York: Simon and Schuster.
It's SARK...need I say more?

Tuesdays With Morrie: An Old Man, a Young Man, and Life's Greatest Lesson by Mitch Albom. (1997). New York: Doubleday.
Bring tissues – this book is fabulous.

Women's Bodies, Women's Wisdom: Creating Physical and Emotional Health and Healing by Christiane Northrup. (1998). New York: Bantam Books.
Beyond a medical model, this is an encyclopedia for women who know there's something more...

Selected Websites

Anxiety Disorders Association of America
www.adaa.org

Anxiety Disorders Association of Canada
www.anxietycanada.ca

The Anxiety Network International
www.anxietynetwork.com

American Psychological Association
About panic disorder:
www.apa.org/pubinfo/panic.html

Anxiety treatment centers in Canada:
www.macanxiety.com/satsc.htm

National Anxiety Foundation
www.lexington-on-line.com/naf.html

National Institute of Mental Health
  1) About Anxiety Disorders:
  www.nimh.nih.gov/healthinformation/anxietymenu.cfm
  2) About Panic Disorder:
  www.nimh.nih.gov/HealthInformation/panicmenu.cfm
  3) Anxiety Community:
  www.healthyplace.com/Communities/Anxiety/nimh/index.asp

National Mental Health Association:
www.nmha.org/pbedu/anxiety/panic.cfm

Thank Yous

To my family...
Nick – Your love allows me to be so much more than I ever imagined. **Mom** – What can I say? There are no words to thank a Mom...they will never do. **Joe** – Generous beyond comprehension, loving beyond measure. **Matthew** – Did you know that you would become an amazingly spiritual person? I love you, little brother! **Rafi** – California loves you! Thanks for San Diego, and San Diego again. "I could live here!" **Dad** – For your love, for your wisdom. "It's only money. You can always make money." **Mom and Dad Pedota** – Thanks always for the soul food. And thanks for Nick.

To my friends...
(too many to thank, please know I love and appreciate you all)
Howie – You were always there. I know that. **Keira** – For massages and great conversations. You are SO smart. **Jen** – Best friends will always be best friends, eh? I love you! **Sun** – Your love and energy are unparalleled. **Stephen** – Thank you for your spirit – you are a mensch. **Vivian** – Thanks for allowing (and forcing) me to put my health first, and my job second. **Sam** – Sam, Sam, Sam! I don't know anyone as unique as you are. I am honoured to be your friend. **Tamara** – What a great inscription...you were right! **Vito** – I thank you for being my friend and making me feel like I am not alone (and for the skate). And for making Nick laugh. **Margie** – If we could all have teachers as sweet and insightful and supportive as you, the world would be a lovelier place. **Norm** – It was fate I walked into your workshop in Toronto. Thank you for your email support, for Joan, and for bringing me to my safe place. **Clare** – I have never met anyone so willing to fight for my rights to take care of my health and to graduate. Thanks, and keep it up! **Ilyse** – For all your emails and cyber-support.

You're awesome! **Cathy Cae** – I am honoured to grow with you day by day, I am honoured to be your friend and to learn from your experiences. Thanks for saving me when I asked for some saving.

To my healers...

Dr. S. – For being my first therapist, and for knowing most people are not really sick (in the body). **Diego** – You are a tireless healer. Thank you for all your support at the beginning. **Lisa** – Thanks for the relaxing massages. The work you do is so important. **Dr. Katz** – Thanks for hitting the nail on the head. **Laurel** – Thank you for your hours and hours of support. We make a great team. We made my recovery possible. **Ken** – Thanks for creating such a warm environment in your practice. Your instincts are usually right. You go beyond the definition of chiropractor. **Dr. Simpson** – If only all M.D.'s could be like you. **Michella** – It's great to have a massage therapist who is also a friend. What talented hands. **Riki** – For your support during my first year of teaching. **Connie** – Thank you for your loving support and prayer. You are making a difference. **Tunde** – For your insightful Reiki sessions and healing hands. **Marco** – What a talented Shiatsu therapist. Intuitive, amazing. **Darby** – Thanks for reminding me that I always have a choice. **Billy** – You are a gifted healer, and wonderful person. Thanks for asking to see the book.

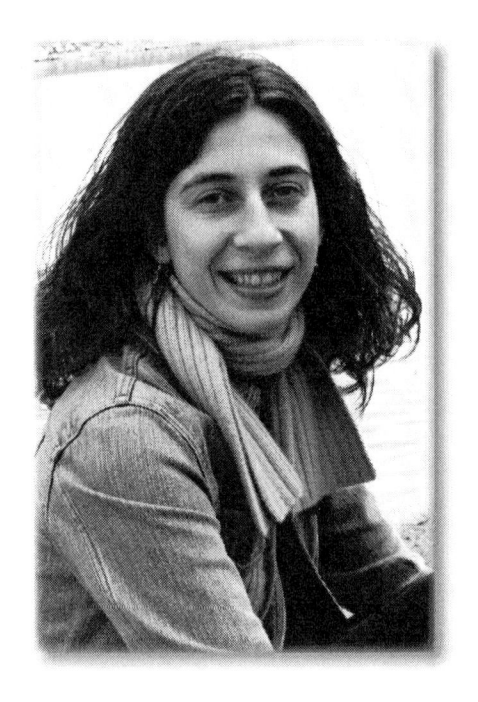

Bonnie Grzesh Pedota is a speaker, writer and educator. She is studying to become a Spiritual Psychotherapist. Bonnie's great joys include giggling with her husband Nick, visiting mountains, lakes and oceans, and nurturing her Spirit. Bonnie looks forward to her next writing adventure.

To book a speaking engagement or to contact Bonnie,
please email bonnie@bonsyearon.com.

www.bonsyearon.com

ISBN 1-41206439-2